Low Fodmap Diet Cookbook For Beginners

1500 Days of Simple and Healthy Recipes For Improving Your IBS & Digestive Disorders to Make Your Gut Happier

BY

DONNA JOHNSON

TABLE OF CONTENTS

INTRODUCTION

You may have heard of the FODMAP diet via a friend or on the internet. When people mention "FODMAP diet," they typically imply a diet low in FODMAP – specific sugars that may cause intestinal irritation. This diet is meant to assist persons with irritable bowel syndrome (IBS) and/or small intestinal bacterial overgrowth (SIBO) find out which meals are troublesome and which foods alleviate symptoms.

The low FODMAP diet is a temporary eating plan that's very restrictive. It's always good to talk to your doctor before starting a new diet, but especially with the low FODMAP diet since it eliminates so many foods, it's not a diet anyone should follow for long. It's a quick discovery procedure to identify what meals are bothersome for you. In this cookbook, we will explore the basics of the FODMAP Diet and provide you with a variety of delicious and easy-to-make recipes that are low in FODMAPs. Whether you are new to the FODMAP Diet or have been following it for a while, this cookbook will serve as a valuable resource for creating flavorful and satisfying meals that won't aggravate your digestive system.

What is Irritable Bowel Syndrome?

Irritable bowel syndrome (IBS) is a functional disorder that affects 11% of the worldwide population. About 30% of the individuals who suffer symptoms don't contact a doctor but rather understand what is feasible from internet publications and implement a few basic modifications to their diets to settle on a solution that works.

Everything you consume might have an influence on your body. In rare situations, it might create digestive troubles or exasperate your IBS. By consuming low FODMAP foods, decreasing these responses to bearable levels or eliminating them is feasible.

What are Fodmaps

What does FODMAP stand for, exactly?

Fermentable: Fermentable carbohydrates are carbohydrates that are broken down by intestinal bacteria through fermentation. The fermentation process of digestion contrasts with enzymatic digestion, which does not cause much gas or intestinal discomfort.

Oligosaccharide: Oligosaccharides are carbohydrates formed when three to six units of simple sugars (monosaccharides) share bonds.

Disaccharide: A disaccharide is the sugar generated when two monosaccharides share bonds.

Monosaccharide: Monosaccharides (fructose), often termed simple sugars, are sugars in their simplest forms.

Polyols: Polyols are hydrogenated monosaccharides and include foods like apples, cherries, pears, and plums.

Why do Fodmaps Cause Gas

In brief, these short-chain carbohydrates, while moving through the small intestine, tend to depend largely on bacteria fermentation which via osmosis sucks water into the colon, creating all sorts of pain.

Fermentation occurs when the small intestine is not capable of breaking down the carbohydrates. As a consequence, the FODMAP meal will find its way to the end of the gut, meet its match, bacteria.

In other words, FODMAPs are short-chain carbohydrates that typically resist digestion. These carbs are present naturally in various meals and affect everyone differently.

The quantity of gas generated as the result of bacterial digestion is based on how much FODMAP meal needs bacteria intervention to break down.

Types of Fodmaps

There are five primary kinds of FODMAPs.

1. Fructose
Fructose is a simple sugar. It's present in high fructose corn syrup, fruits, honey, and vegetables. Foods that contain fructose include:

- Agave syrup
- Honey
- Most juices
- Grapes Peas Zucchini Apples

2. Lactose Lactose is a carb present in dairy products like milk. Though not all persons with IBS are lactose intolerant, it might make IBS symptoms worse.

Foods tend to differ in lactose content, however. While certain lactose-containing meals may produce symptoms, others might not.

Foods that contain lactose include:
- Cow and goat milk
- Ice cream
- Cheese Yogurt
- Baked foods with milk

3. Fructans

Fructans are non-digestible carbohydrates. They're present in barley, rye, wheat, and spelt. They're also present in veggies like onions and garlic.

When gut bacteria attack fructans, it initiates a fermentation process. This fermentation may give some health advantages. However, it might also produce undesirable IBS symptoms.

Foods that contain fructans include:

- Wheat Barley
- Rye Garlic Onions
- Cashews
- Watermelon
- Asparagus Bananas

4. Galactooligosaccharides

Also known as galactans or GOS. This carb is found in legumes including chickpeas, lentils, and beans. Like fructans, galactans are non-digestible and may consequently induce IBS difficulties.

Foods that contain galactans include:

- Soy products
- Lentils Beans
- Pistachios Oat milk
- Lentils

5. Polyols Polyols are sugar alcohols that commonly end in "-tol." A few include maltitol, mannitol, xylitol, and sorbitol. Some polys appear naturally in fruits and vegetables like blackberries and mushrooms.

Polys are also utilized as artificial sweeteners.

Foods that contain polys include:

- Cauliflower Stone fruits

- Avocado
- Blackberries
- Corn Celery
- Sweet potatoes
- Mushrooms
- Artificial sweeteners

If you have IBS, you may not discover that you're sensitive to every kind of FODMAP. With that in mind, the FODMAP diet involves an elimination approach. You'll remove every form of FODMAP, then re-introduce one at a time.

The methodical procedure helps you to establish which foods trigger your symptoms. Then, you may preserve the things you tolerate well inside your diet.

Before following this approach, be sure you talk with a doctor or competent dietary expert. They may make sure you finish the procedure with your health in mind. A misdiagnosis of IBS due to FODMAPs with Irritable Bowel Disorder (IBD) is no little error.

How do Fodmaps Affect the Body

What precisely occurs when you consume FODMAP diet foods?

Many FODMAPs will pass through the bulk of your gut without experiencing alterations. FODMAPs are digestion-resistant.

For certain individuals, carbohydrates work like FODMAPs, such as fructose and lactose. Sensitivity might vary between persons. If you're sensitive to a certain FODMAP, it might create stomach difficulties.

Once the FODMAP enters your colon, the fermentation process starts. Then, your gut bacteria will utilize the fermented FODMAP for energy. This is the same procedure your body completes to feed favorable gut microorganisms.

Positive gut flora helps avoid health disorders including irritable bowel syndrome, diarrhea, and eczema.

Friendly gut microorganisms may create methane. Bacteria from FODMAPs, on the other hand, create both hydrogen and methane which might cause you to suffer discomfort, constipation, stomach cramps, gas, distention, and bloating.

Since FODMAPs are osmotically active, they may suck water into the colon producing diarrhea and dehydration.

Who Should Use the FODMAP Diet?

Many individuals with IBS experience a range of symptoms, with around 40% having mild symptoms, 35% experiencing moderate instances, and 25% dealing with severe IBS. It's important to note that some people may not even realize they have IBS. Here are some potential signs to keep an eye out for:

- Pain and cramping
- Diarrhea
- Constipation
- Alternating constipation and diarrhea
- Fatigue
- Difficulting sleeping
- Anxiety and depression
- Bowel movement changes

- Gas and bloating
- Food intolerance

About 70% of persons with IBS claim certain meals cause their symptoms. Unfortunately, there's no well-defined etiology for IBS. Many individuals think food and stress may both have an influence.

Switching to the low-FODMAP diet might ease your IBS symptoms. Reducing your symptoms might improve your quality of life.

In fact, adopting a low FODMAP diet food list might assist people with various functional gastrointestinal diseases (FGID). It might also aid individuals with inflammatory bowel illnesses, such as ulcerative colitis and Crohn's disease.

If the low-FODMAP diet works for you, you could experience less:

- Stomach pain
- Constipation
- Diarrhea
- Bloating Gas

Remember, everyone responds to FODMAPs differently. How the low-FODMAP diet impacts you might vary from someone else's experience. Keep an open mind and stay realistic before consuming low-FODMAP diet items.

Switching to a low-FODMAP diet might have a psychological advantage, too. Many intestinal disorders may cause stress and humiliation. In certain circumstances, irritable bowel syndrome is associated with anxiety and depression as well.

50% to 90% of the persons who seek therapy for IBS have psychological issues. These include serious depression, PTSD, social phobia, panic disorder, and generalized anxiety disorder. Scientists are constantly discovering more about how the gut-brain link works.

By switching to a low-FODMAP diet, you might lessen your anxiety and sadness.

Steps to Prepare for the Low Fodmap Diet

If you intend on following the low-FODMAP diet, you'll need to finish each level. Here are the three steps of an efficient FODMAP diet.

Restriction

First, you'll need to eliminate any high-FODMAP foods. Remove these items from your diet for three to eight weeks. Instead, concentrate on your low-FODMAP diet food list.

Do you detect any difference in your gut health? Are you having IBS symptoms less often? If it seems like your gut health has improved, you may continue on to the next phase.

Reintroduction

You may now start incorporating high-FODMAP foods back into your diet. The reintroduction step will help you identify which FODMAPs you can tolerate. You'll also utilize this step to establish your threshold level. Your threshold reflects the quantity of FODMAPs your body can handle.

During the reintroduction stage, you'll try each meal one by one, for three days at a time. Consider consulting with a certified dietician throughout this procedure. You'll continue consuming low-FODMAP diet items throughout the reintroduction phase.

Personalization

Once you've finished the reintroduction step, you should know which FODMAP foods you can and can't consume. Now, you may go onto the customizing step. This stage is also termed the modified low-FODMAP diet.

In this step, you'll still need to block certain high-FODMAPs. You could have noticed that low-FODMAP meals cause your IBS, too. Using what you learnt in the previous step, you'll tailor your diet with your tolerance levels in mind. Consider the quantity and kind of each FODMAP you tolerated. You may incorporate these items to your regimen immediately!

This step will help you stay flexible with your diet. It may also help you add more diversity to what you consume. Following your tailored FODMAP diet may enhance your quality of life and digestive health long-term.

If your symptoms don't improve, be sure to evaluate the items you're consuming. Look for ingredient lists to locate high-FODMAPs. Then, eliminate these foods.

Consider the pressures in your life, too. Even if you make modifications to your diet, stress might still increase your IBS symptoms.

Remember, everyone responds to FODMAP foods differently.
Keep it in mind as you begin this procedure.

How does the low FODMAP diet work?

Before you transition to a low-FODMAP diet, it is best to know which items to add to your diet and which foods to avoid. Remember, the FODMAP diet works via an elimination phase. You'll eliminate all high FODMAP items from your diet initially.

It is best to follow the elimination component of the diet for approximately two to six weeks.
Then, you'll progressively put meals back into your regimen to observe which ones produce gastrointestinal discomfort.

First, let's speak about the things you should include in your diet. This low-FODMAP diet food list might help you get started.

Make sure to incorporate lots of fish, meats, and eggs to your diet. These meals are typically well-tolerated. Check the label to be sure these items don't include FODMAP elements like high-fructose corn syrup or wheat.

When cooking, experiment with various fats and oils. For example, you may add olive oil to your next recipe. Olive oil is abundant in omega-3 fatty acids, which give health advantages such

- Improving eye health
- Fighting anxiety and sadness
- Fighting inflammation (which is related with heart disease, cancer, and other illnesses)
- Promoting brain health during pregnancy
- Alleviating menstruation pain
- Improving sleep Reducing ADHD symptoms in children
- Improving the condition of your skin (cutting the risk of acne and premature aging)
- Reducing the risk of some malignancies
- Fighting autoimmune disorders (multiple sclerosis, type 1 diabetes, Crohn's disease, etc.)

- Reducing metabolic syndrome symptoms
- Reducing asthma in children and young adults
- Improving mental diseases (bipolar disorder, schizophrenia, etc.)
- Fighting age-related deterioration and Alzheimer's
- Reducing fat in the liver
- Improving bone and joint health
- Improving risk factors for heart disease

As you cook, add additional spices and herbs into the mix, too. Herbs and spices may transform a plain food into a tasty delight.

Try to incorporate nuts and seeds among your low FODMAP diet items, including:

- Sesame seeds
- Peanuts
- Cashews Almonds
- Macadamia nuts
- Pine nuts

There are many fruits you can consume that aren't heavy in fructose. For example, you may include blueberries, grapefruit, lemons, oranges, and strawberries to your diet.

There are low-FODMAP sweeteners you can use, too. Consider utilizing molasses, stevia, and maple syrup to substitute sugar alcohols.

Remember, there are certain sources of lactose you can consume, including hard cheese. Consider matured, softer cheeses like camembert and brie, too. Otherwise, try switching to lactose-free dairy products.

You can still consume veggies on a low-FODMAP diet, too! These veggies include:
- Bell peppers Bok choy Carrots
- Cucumbers
- Green beans
- Kale
- Lettuce
- Spanish Potatoes

You can also consume grains including quinoa, rice, oats, and maize.

Remember, everyone responds to FODMAPs differently.

The elimination diet will help you develop a FODMAP diet that's perfect for you.

Food to Avoid and Food to Enjoy

If you are following a low FODMAP diet, it's crucial to know which items are safe to consume and which ones to avoid. Low FODMAP foods are those that have minimum quantities of fermentable carbohydrates that might cause digestive symptoms in persons with irritable bowel syndrome (IBS) and other digestive problems. By including a range of low FODMAP foods in your diet, you can ensure that you are obtaining the nutrients you need while also controlling your symptoms. In this part, we will discuss some of the finest low FODMAP foods to include in your diet and the high FODMAP foods you should avoid.

High FODMAP meals that you should avoid include:

Fructose: Fruits (including apples, mangos, pears, melons), honey, high-fructose corn syrup, agave

Lactose: Dairy (milk from cows, goats, or sheep), custard, yogurt, ice cream

Fructans: Rye and Wheat, asparagus, broccoli, cabbage, onions, garlic

Galactans: Legumes, such as beans (particularly baked beans), lentils, chickpeas, and soybeans

Polyols: Sugar alcohols and fruits that include pits or seeds, such as apples, apricots, avocados, cherries, figs, peaches, pears, or plums

Low FODMAP meals to enjoy instead include:
Dairy: Almond milk, lactose-free milk, rice milk, coconut milk, lactose-free yogurt, and hard cheeses.

Fruit: Bananas, blueberries, cantaloupe, grapefruit, honeydew, kiwi, lemon, lime, oranges, and strawberries.

Vegetables: Bamboo shoots, bean sprouts, bok choy, carrots, chives, cucumbers, eggplant, ginger, lettuce, olives, parsnips, potatoes, spring onions, and turnips.

Protein: Beef, pig, poultry, fish, eggs, and tofu.

Nuts/seeds: (limit to 10-15 each) Almonds, macadamia nuts, peanuts, pine nuts, and walnuts.

Grain: Oats, oat bran, rice bran, gluten-free pasta, quinoa, white rice, and corn flour.

Benefits of Fodmap

In one study, 66% of the patients who followed a reduced FODMAP diet were satisfied with their symptom control. All symptoms (bloating, abdominal pain, flatulence, tiredness) improved with the reduced FODMAP diet.

The low-FODMAP diet isn't for everyone, though. If your doctor hasn't diagnosed you with IBS, switching to low FODMAP diet items could negatively affect your gut health.

Why? Most FODMAPs are prebiotics. Prebiotics support healthy microorganisms in your gut.

We need prebiotics to protect our bodies from dangerous microbes. Good gut flora could increase your immune system functions. They could help with weight and depression, too.

Some gut bacteria even help create vitamin K and short-chain fatty acids, which promote a stronger gut barrier. This barrier protects the intestines from viruses, germs, and inflammation.

In fact, short-chain fatty acids could even lessen your risk of cancer.
The FODMAP diet is suitable for anyone who has ongoing digestive issues and hasn't responded to first-line dietary guidance. It can also help if you haven't responded to stress management measures.

Here are a few perks you might enjoy by adopting the FODMAP diet.

Reduces digestive symptoms: FODMAPs are short-chain carbohydrates that are poorly absorbed by the small intestine. When they reach the colon, they are fermented by bacteria, which may induce gas, bloating, diarrhea, and constipation. A low-FODMAP diet may help to decrease these symptoms by decreasing the consumption of FODMAP-rich foods.

Improves quality of life: Digestive issues may have a substantial influence on quality of life. A low-FODMAP diet may assist to enhance quality of life by lowering digestive symptoms and enabling patients to engage in activities that they may have previously avoided due to their symptoms.

Improves IBS symptoms: Irritable bowel syndrome (IBS) is a persistent digestive illness that affects millions of individuals worldwide. A low-FODMAP diet has been demonstrated to be useful in lowering IBS symptoms, such as stomach discomfort, bloating, diarrhea, and constipation.

Improves SIBO symptoms: Small intestinal bacterial overgrowth (SIBO) is a disorder in which there is an excessive quantity of bacteria in the small intestine. SIBO may produce digestive symptoms, such as bloating, gas, diarrhea, and stomach discomfort. A low-FODMAP diet may assist to reduce SIBO symptoms by lowering the quantity of food that is available for bacteria to ferment.

Improves gastrointestinal health: FODMAPs may nourish harmful microorganisms in the stomach. A low-FODMAP diet may assist to enhance gut health by limiting the quantity of FODMAPs available to feed bad bacteria.

Improves nutrition absorption: FODMAPs may interfere with the absorption of nutrients from meals. A low-FODMAP diet may assist to increase nutrient absorption by lowering the quantity of FODMAPs in the diet.

Improves mental health: Digestive issues may have a detrimental influence on mental health. A low-FODMAP diet may assist to promote mental health by lowering digestive symptoms and enhancing quality of life.

Reduced inflammation: FODMAPs may promote inflammation in the digestive system. This inflammation may lead to digestive problems, such as stomach discomfort, bloating, and diarrhea. A low-FODMAP diet may assist to decrease inflammation in the digestive system and alleviate digestive symptoms.

Improved energy levels: Digestive problems may sap energy levels. A low-FODMAP diet may assist to increase energy levels by minimizing digestive discomfort and enhancing nutrition absorption.

Low-FODMAP Diet Advice

Following the low-FODMAP diet is a hard task. Before you get started, no your doctor could urge you to adopt first-line methods. Below is a selection of common practices you may consider addressing with your physician.

Eat Regularly: First, develop a timetable for regular, consistent meals. Eating often will guarantee you're not overeating in one sitting. Sometimes, overeating might worsen IBS symptoms.

Get Enough Fiber: You'll need fiber to boost your gastrointestinal and colon health.
If you're suffering from diarrhea, consider meals containing soluble fiber. These include squash, carrots, oats, and chia seeds.

If you're battling with constipation, obtain a combination of soluble and insoluble fiber. Insoluble fiber includes fruits, vegetables, brown rice, quinoa, nuts, and seeds.

Remove Irritants: Consider becoming purposeful with the elimination of irritants from your diet that can damage your digestive health. These include alcohol, energy drinks, caffeine, and spicy meals.

Avoid High-Fat Meals: High-fat diets might aggravate your IBS symptoms owing to the inherent inclination of fats to increase intestinal contractions.

Avoid Sweeteners: Check the labels on your favorite foods and check for sugar alcohols, high fructose corn syrup, fructose, or honey.

Manage Your Stress: Remember, the gut-brain link might induce IBS symptoms. Try to regulate your stress levels. Consider taking up yoga or meditation for a spell.

Equipment for Fodmap

When it comes to creating low FODMAP meals, having the correct equipment and supplies may make all the difference. Here are some necessary kitchen utensils and items for a low FODMAP diet:

1. chopping board: Use a separate chopping board for fruits and vegetables that are rich in FODMAPs to prevent cross-contamination.

2. Knife set: A nice pair of knives will help you effortlessly cut and prepare your low FODMAP items.

3. Vegetable peeler: This equipment is useful for peeling vegetables including carrots, zucchini, and potatoes.

4. Measuring cups and spoons: Accurate measuring of ingredients is vital for low FODMAP cooking.

5. Non-stick frying pan: A non-stick pan will let you cook without using additional fats or oils.

6. making sheet: Perfect for roasting low FODMAP veggies or making gluten-free bread or pastries.

Tips on Eating Out

Eating out on a low FODMAP diet might seem scary, but with the appropriate methods and advice, you can easily enjoy meals outside the home.

One of the finest things you can do while dining out is to conduct some homework before you get to the restaurant. Here are some ways you may prepare ahead to make low FODMAP eating out less stressful.

Before You Arrive at the Restaurant

Check out the menu online: Luckily, it's now simpler than ever to check out a restaurant's menu online before you go. Take a look at the menu and make a note of any items that appear like they'll work for you. Once you arrive at the restaurant, you may check with the serving personnel that the dish doesn't contain any high FODMAP items.

Call ahead: If you cannot locate menu information online, consider phoning the restaurant ahead to ask if they can accommodate low FODMAP selections. Restaurants enjoy being advised in advance that they may need to make adjustments to fit your dietary preferences, and this may bring peace of mind that you'll be able to dine at the restaurant.

Consider eateries that provide gluten-free choices: While gluten isn't technically the issue on a low FODMAP diet, gluten-free alternatives are also wheat-free. Since wheat is a big source of FODMAPs, selecting gluten-free choices may be a simple move to guarantee your meal is low FODMAP. Try finding eateries that provide a good selection of gluten-free foods.

Consider eating during off-peak hours: If possible, try to eat during periods when the restaurant is not as crowded. This will make it easy to communicate with the waitress about your dietary preferences and will guarantee the kitchen has adequate time to prepare your dish.

Bring a written list of items you need to avoid: Communication is crucial, and having a list of things you need to avoid may be quite beneficial for the restaurant staff. Try to bring a written list of the items you need to avoid so that your waiter may submit it to the chef and ensure that no high FODMAP components are added to your meal.

At the Restaurant

Once you're in the restaurant, try to pick dishes that can be readily altered to be low FODMAP. Here are some sorts of meals that are normally safe to order or can be simply changed to be low FODMAP.

Grilled or roasted chicken, beef, pig, or seafood: Grilled meats are frequently good alternatives for low FODMAP dining out. Be cautious to inquire if the meat has been marinated or seasoned with high FODMAP items like onion and garlic. If it has, ask if they can make the protein without these components. Pair with a side of steamed veggies and a carbohydrate like rice, quinoa, or potatoes for a full meal.

Salads: Salads are often simple to modify to your dietary needs. Many dressings include garlic, so ask if they can season the salad with lemon juice or vinegar and olive oil instead (or bring your own dressing to use!). When ordering a salad, watch out for high FODMAP foods such croutons and dried berries.

Pizza: Choose a gluten-free pizza base with simple tomato paste. Top the pizza with low FODMAP components and suggest that they do not add any high FODMAP elements like onion or garlic to the toppings or sauce.

Sushi: Many varieties of sushi are inherently low FODMAP. If you order rolls with avocado, restrict your portion amount, since avocado is high FODMAP in serving sizes of ¼ avocado or greater. You may also want to minimize any rolls that include tempura, since tempura is prepared with wheat flour, which is high FODMAP. The little quantity of wheat included in soy sauce normally isn't a concern for someone following the low FODMAP diet.

Pasta: Many restaurants will provide a gluten-free alternative for their pasta meals. Be cautious to check if the spices and sauce include high FODMAP items such onion, garlic, and cream, and ask if these elements may be avoided.

Keep your non-FODMAP IBS triggers in mind
While it's feasible to find low FODMAP choices while eating out, it's crucial to note that FODMAPs are not the main source of symptoms for those with IBS. Some of the potential causes for IBS symptoms include:
- High-fat meals
- Spicy food
- Alcohol Caffeine

Try to be cautious of these additional IBS triggers to ensure you're not mistakenly consuming non-FODMAP foods that might induce symptoms.

Measurements Conversion Chart

Measurement	Conversion
1 teaspoon (tsp)	5 milliliters (ml)
1 tablespoon (Thsp)	15 milliliters (ml)
1 fluid ounce (fl oz)	30 milliliters (ml)
1 cup	240 milliliters (ml)/8 fluid ounces (fl oz)

1 pint (pt)	2 cups/480 milliliters (ml)/16 fluid ounces (fl oz)
1 quart (gt)	2 pints (pt)/32 fluid ounces (fl oz)/0.946 liters (1)
1 gallon (gal)	4 quarts (qt)/128 fluid ounces (fl ez)/3.785 liters (1)
1 ounce (n)	28.35 grams (g)
1 pound (lb)	16 ounces (or)/454 grams (g)
1. kilogram (kg)	2.204 pounds (lb)/35.27 ounces (oz)

Temperature Conversion Chart

Fahrenheit (°F)	Celsius (°C)
30°F	0°C
50°F	10°C
68°F	20°C
86°F	30°C
104°F	40°C

122°F	50°C
140°F	60°C
158°F	70°C
176°F	80°C
194°F	90°C
212°F	100°C

BREAKFAST RECIPES

Low-FODMAP Breakfast Casserole

Servings size: 14   Prep Time: 5 minutes
Cook Time: 1 hour   Total Time: 1 hour 5 mins

INGREDIENTS:
- 24- ounce to 30-ounce (680 g to 685 g) container of low FODMAP frozen hash browns, roughly 8 to 9 cups
- 1- pound (455 g) thickly sliced low FODMAP ham, diced 8- ounces (225 g) sharp cheddar cheese, shredded 12 big eggs
- 1 cup (240 ml) lactose-free whole milk
- Kosher salt
- Freshly ground black pepper

INSTRUCTIONS
1. Position rack in center of oven.
2. Preheat the oven to 350°C (180°C).
3. Coat the interior of a 13-inch by 9-inch (33 cm by 23 cm) casserole dish with nonstick spray; set aside.

4. Toss together the frozen hash browns, ham and cheese in a large basin to thoroughly blend, then scrape into the prepared pan, producing an equal layer.

5. In the same basin, mix the eggs and milk until fully incorporated. Season with salt and pepper, then pour evenly over the potato mixture. Gently pat everything down with the back of a sturdy spoon.

6. Bake for one hour, uncovered or until the center is set and the sides are golden brown. Let sit for 5 minutes and serve.

TIPS

- I like to offer low FODMAP spicy sauce or salsa alongside. Some people prefer ketchup with their eggs, and since there are low FODMAP portion sizes, why not provide it? We have an excellent essay about Condiments, by the way

NUTRITION VALUE

Calories: 216 kcal | Carbs: 12g | Protein: 15g | Fat: 17g | Sodium: 151mg

Overnight Oats With Chocolate and Strawberries

Servings size: 1
Total Time: 8 hours 5 mins

INGREDIENTS

- ⅓ cup rolled oats (use gluten-free rolled oats for gluten-free)
- ½ cup unsweetened almond milk (or other low FODMAP milk)
- 1 tbsp chia seeds
- 2 tablespoons pure maple syrup
- 1 teaspoon unsweetened cocoa powder
- 2 big strawberries
- 2 teaspoon Enjoy Life Mini Chocolate Chips, optional

INSTRUCTIONS

1. Place oats, milk, chia seeds, maple syrup, and cocoa powder into a sealable container and whisk to incorporate (or cover and shake – my favorite option!). If it isn't already, cover oats and store in the fridge overnight (or for at least two hours).

2. Right before serving, dice strawberries. Give the oats a quick swirl and sprinkle with strawberries and optional chocolate chips. Serve chilled.

NOTES

- Rolled Oats: A low FODMAP serving is up to a ½ cup or 52 grams.

- Chia Seeds: A low FODMAP serving is up to 2 tablespoons or 24 grams.

- Cocoa Powder: A low FODMAP serving is up to 2 heaped tablespoons or 8 grams.

NUTRITION VALUE
Calories Per Serving: 300 % 11%Total Fat 8.5g 17%Total Carbohydrate 45.9g 34%Dietary Fiber 9.6g 16%Protein 8g

---

Strata Of Ham And Cheese

Servings size: 16   Prep Time 15 mins
Time to cook: 40 mins Total Time: 55 mins

INGREDIENTS

- 10 big eggs that are room temperature
- 2 cups (480 ml) of lactose-free milk or half-and-half, like Organic Valley
- 2 tablespoons of Dijon mustard
- You can add either 1/2 teaspoon of dried thyme or 1 teaspoon of fresh Kosher salt.
- Ground black pepper just now
- 4 cups (225 g) cubed low FODMAP, gluten-free French bread
- 8 ounces (225 g) ham, chopped, such as from our Brown Sugar Baked Ham
- 8 ounces (225 g) shredded cheese, such as cheddar, Gruyere, Monterey Jack or a mix
- 1/2 dry pint (275 g) fresh tomatoes, split

INSTRUCTIONS:

1. Whisk together the eggs very well in a big bowl with milk or half-and-half. Whisk in mustard and thyme and season with salt and pepper. Note that the cheese and ham bring a lot of salt to the mix. I often make this layer without salt, so at the very least use a light hand. But definitely do add black pepper, which adds balance to the dish. Fold in cubed

bread and allow to sit while you warm the oven.

2. Position rack in middle of oven.

3. Preheat the oven to 350°F/180°C. Coat the inside of a 13 x 9-inch (33 cm x 23 cm) baking dish with nonstick spray.

4. Fold ham, cheeses and veggies into strata mixture and scrape into prepared pan.

5. Bake for about 35 to 45 minutes or until custard is set. The layer will puff up a bit and uncovered pieces of bread will get crispy here and there, which is great. Cool pan on a rack for 5 minutes and serve warm or at room temperature. The strata can be refrigerated but should be warmed at least up to room temperature, which you can do in the microwave or a low oven.

6. TIPS You do have choices when it comes to the cheese component. You need a good soft cheese, such as those listed. A mix is often nice. I do like to use the Gruyere, which I especially love with ham, and pair it with cheese.

NUTRITION

Calories: 163 kcal | Carbohydrates: 7g | Protein: 12g | Fat: 10g | Saturated Fat: 1g | Cholesterol: 132 mg | Sodium: 189 mg | Potassium: 49mg | Fiber: 1g | Sugar: 2g | Calcium: 20mg | Iron: 0.6mg

---

Spinach + Feta Tofu Scramble

Servings size: 3   *Prep Time: 5 Mins*
Cook Time: 10 Mins   *Total Time: 15 Mins*

INGREDIENTS

- 1 tablespoon avocado oil
- 1 package extra-firm tofu, patted dry
- ½ cup green onion, green tops only, thinly sliced
- 2 tsp healthy yeast
- ½ + ⅛ teaspoon salt
- ½ teaspoon ground cumin
- ½ teaspoon turmeric
- ½ teaspoon dried thyme
- freshly cracked pepper
- 4 big handfuls baby spinach, roughly chopped ½ cup vegan feta cheese, crumbled

- If NOT low FODMAP, add ½ teaspoon onion powder

INSTRUCTIONS

1. Add avocado oil to a nonstick pan on medium heat. Crumble tofu into a pan, and sprinkle it with green onions, nutritional yeast, salt, cumin, turmeric, thyme and pepper.
2. Cook, stirring occasionally, until cooked through and getting a bit browned, about 4-5 minutes.
3. Add spinach and ⅓ cup (75 mL) water, and heat, turning often, until spinach is wilted and water is mostly drained, about 2 minutes. Turn off heat and stir in vegan feta cheese.
4. Serve with a slice of sprouted grain or sourdough toast for a full and rewarding breakfast

NUTRITION

Calories: 163 kcal | Carbohydrates: 7g | Protein: 12g | Fat: 10g | Saturated Fat: 1g | Cholesterol: 132 mg | Sodium: 189 mg | Potassium: 49mg | Fiber: 1g | Sugar: 2g | Calcium: 20mg | Iron: 0.6mg

Low Fodmap Breakfast Pork Sausage Patties

Serving Size :8 Prep Time: 5 mins
Cook Time: 10 mins. Total Time: 15 mins

INGREDIENTS:
- 1 tablespoon tightly packed light brown sugar
- 1 tablespoon finely chopped fresh sage or 1 teaspoon rubbed (ground) sage
- 1 tablespoon finely chopped fresh thyme or 1 teaspoon dried thyme
- 11/4 teaspoons kosher salt
- 1 teaspoon crushed fennel seeds
- ½ teaspoon chili powder, such as ground red serrano chili
- ¼ teaspoon paprika
- Freshly Ground black pepper
- 1 pound (455 g) ground pork

INSTRUCTIONS
1. Place brown sugar, sage, thyme, salt, fennel seeds, chili and paprika in a medium sized mixing bowl. Add a large amount of black pepper. Use your fingers to rub the mixture together to make sure all the herbs and spices are well mixed. Add the pork and mix

everything together well. (This mixture can be made the night ahead, if you are planning a big start. Just cover the bowl with plastic wrap).

2. Use a 1/4-cup (60 ml) measuring cup or similar sized ice cream scoop to make cakes, pressed to about 1/4-inch (6 mm) thick. They will increase in thickness upon cooking.

3. Heat a cast iron or heavy pan over medium-high heat. Cook patties for about 2 to 3 minutes or until golden brown on bottom, flip and cook second side until golden. The patties should be cooked through.

4. Sausages are ready to serve. They may also be frozen: cool first, stack in single layers divided by parchment paper in a sealed container and freeze for up to 1 month. You can heat them on the stovetop in a pan or in the microwave.

NUTRITION

Calories: 155 kcal | Carbohydrates: 2g | Protein: 10g | Fat: 12g | Saturated Fat: 4g | Cholesterol: 41mg | Sodium: 831 mg | Potassium: 163 mg | Sugar: 1g | Calcium: 8mg

Low Fodmap Quinoa, Greens & Bell Pepper Puff

Servings size: 6 *Prep Time: 10 minutes*
Cook Time: 40 mins *Total Time: 50 minutes*

INGREDIENTS

- 10 ounces (280 g) Swiss chard 5 ounces (140 g) baby spinach
- 2 teaspoons Garlic-Infused Oil, produced using olive oil, or bought equivalent
- 1/2 cup (36 g) finely sliced leeks, green parts only
- 1/2 cup (32 g) freshly cut scallions, green parts only
- 1/2 red bell pepper (150 g), cored and diced
- 1/2 teaspoon dried thyme
- Kosher salt
- Freshly ground black pepper
- 6 big eggs, at room temperature
- 3/4 cup (81 g) shredded Gruyere or cheddar cheese
- 1 cup (185 g) cooked quinoa

INSTRUCTIONS

1. Position rack in center of oven. Preheat the oven to 375°F/190°C. Coat the interior of a 1 ½ quart to 2-quart (1.4 L to 2 L) casserole dish with nonstick spray; set aside.

2. Bring a big saucepan of salted water to a boil. Meanwhile, slice off and remove the very ends of the Swiss chard. Finely cut the remaining stalks and leaves. Add all of the Swiss chard and the spinach to the boiling water and boil for a minute or two, stirring all the greens into the water to be fully soaked, simmering until wilted. Drain the colander in the sink and leave to cool.

3. Meanwhile, add oil to a large sauté pan over low-medium heat and heat until shimmering; add leeks, onions and red bell pepper and sauté for a couple of minutes until softened. Season with thyme and generously with salt and pepper.

4. Going back to the colander in the sink, use the back of a heavy spoon to press water out of the greens, then use your hands if required to squeeze as much water out of them as possible. You may wrap them up in a clean tea towel and really wring them out over the

sink. Add to the sauté pan, tossing everything together thoroughly. Taste and adjust seasoning. Cool momentarily.

5. Whisk eggs in a large bowl, whisk in cheese, then add cooled vegetable mixture and cooked quinoa and toss everything together thoroughly. Scrape into the prepared dish and bake for approximately 20 to 25 minutes or until eggs are just set and the mixture is a bit puffed.

NUTRITION

Calories: 245 kcal | Carbohydrates: 15g | Protein: 13g | Fat: 15g | Saturated Fat: 1g | Sodium: 269 mg | Potassium: 379mg | Fiber: 3g | Sugar: 1g | Vitamin A: 5105IU | Vitamin C: 20.8mg | Calcium: 54mg | Iron: 2.2mg

---

Scrambled Eggs With Smoked Salmon & Cream Cheese

Makes: 6 Servings. Prep Time: 5 minutes
Cook Time: 5 minutes. Total Time: 10 minutes

INGREDIENTS

- 12 big eggs, at room temperature
- Kosher salt
- Freshly ground black pepper
- 2 tablespoons unsalted butter
- 8 ounces (225 g) cold-smoked salmon, split or chopped into bite-sized pieces, divided 4 ounces (115 g) lactose-free cream cheese, split, such as Green Valley Organics
- Fresh chives
- Fresh dill

INSTRUCTIONS

1. Whisk eggs very well in a large bowl with a splash of water and season thoroughly with salt and pepper; leave aside.
2. Melt butter in a large, nonstick skillet until foaming over low-medium heat, moving it around to cover the pan bottom and up the sides a little bit.
3. Add the eggs and simmer gently for a minute or two, then begin to move the edges in towards the middle as they begin to set.
4. Dot the top with half of the smoked salmon and half of the cream cheese and continue to

scramble the eggs until they are light and fluffy, but still a touch wet and not dry.

5. Quickly dot the top with leftover smoked salmon and cream cheese, add some clipped chives and fresh dill, to taste, and serve immediately.

NUTRITION

Calories: 311 kcal | Carbohydrates: 2g | Protein: 21g | Fat: 23g | Saturated Fat: 4g | Cholesterol: 422 mg | Sodium: 908mg | Potassium: 156mg | Sugar: 1g | Vitamin A: 695 IU | Calcium: 67mg | Iron: 2mg

---

Low Fodmap Blt Omelet With Blue Cheese

Servings size 2   Prep Time: 5 mins.
Cook Time: 5 mins Total Time: 10 mins

INGREDIENTS

- 4 big eggs
- 2 teaspoons water
- Kosher salt
- Freshly ground black pepper
- 8 cherry or grape tomatoes, halved

- 4 slices of fried crisp bacon, crumbled or diced into bite-sized pieces
- 2 ounces (55 g) crumbled blue cheese (goes excellent with feta, too)
- Handful of tiny lettuces
- 1 tablespoon unsalted butter

INSTRUCTIONS

1. Whisk the eggs very thoroughly in a medium sized mixing dish. Add the water, season with salt and pepper, then add tomatoes, bacon, cheese and lettuce and stir everything together very well.
2. Melt the butter in a big pan (I use nonstick) over medium heat until bubbling. Pour in the omelet mixture and cook over medium heat until the bottom is starting to firm.
3. Use a spatula to pull in the edges of the omelet gently to enable the remaining liquidy areas to flow towards the edges and touch the pan, tilting the pan if required to help the process.
4. Continue to cook until the omelet has a small amount of moisture left to it, but isn't wet, nor unduly dry. Fold one half of the omelet

over onto the other side, slip onto a dish and serve immediately.

NUTRITION

Calories: 301 kcal | Carbohydrates: 2g | Protein: 18g | Fat: 23g | Sodium: 120mg | Sugar: 1g

---

DARK CHOCOLATE WAFFLES

Makes: 12 Servings.   Prep Time: 10 minutes
Cook Time: 15 minutes. Total Time: 25 minutes

INGREDIENTS

- 2 cups (480 ml) lactose-free whole milk, at room temperature
- 2 teaspoons lemon juice
- 1 3/4 cups (254 g) gluten-free all-purpose flour, such as Bob's 1 to 1 Baking Flour
- 1/2 cup (21 g) sprinkled black cocoa
- 1/4 cup (54 g) tightly packed light brown sugar
- 2 tablespoons baking powder; use gluten-free if following a gluten-free diet
- 1 teaspoon baking soda
- 1 teaspoon salt

- 3 big eggs, at room temperature, whisked until well blended
- 1/2 cup (120 ml) canola or vegetable oil
- 1 teaspoon vanilla extract
- Butter maple syrup, and/or confectioner's sugar, optional
- Lactose-free vanilla ice cream, optional
- Heart-shaped cookie cutter, same size as waffles or sharp paring knife
- Melted semisweet or bittersweet chocolate, coarsely chopped, optional

INSTRUCTIONS

For Waffles:

1. Position rack in center of oven. Preheat the oven to 200°F/60°C. Put a rack on a rimmed baking sheet , and put aside.
2. Combine the milk and lemon juice in a measuring cup and leave it to rest for 5 minutes to thicken.
3. Whisk flour, black cocoa powder, brown sugar, baking powder, baking soda, and salt in a large basin. Make a well in the middle of the dry mixture and add the beaten eggs, thickened milk, oil, and vanilla. Whisk

together until the batter is extremely well blended and smooth.

4. Heat a waffle iron until extremely hot; lightly coat with nonstick spray. Working in batches, cook waffles until cooked through. Transfer to a prepared wire rack and keep heated in the oven until ready to serve.

5. Serve waffles with butter and maple syrup or a sprinkle of confectioners' sugar or create ice cream sandwiches!

To Make Ice Cream Sandwiches:
- For every ice cream sandwich you will need two chilled heart shaped waffles, ½ cup (120 ml/66 g) ice cream and ¼ ounce (7 g) of melted dark chocolate.

1. Soften the ice cream a little bit and spoon it out onto a chopping board. Press it down to a thickness of approximately ¾ inch (2 cm). Cut out heart shapes using a cookie cutter the same size as the hearts, or use a paring knife to cut out heart shapes.

2. Use a wide spatula (like a pancake turner) to scoop up each heart and lay on one heart

shaped waffle, topped with a second waffle and gently press together.

3. Smooth the edges of the ice cream, if required, using a little offset spatula. Freeze until firm on a tray or pan.

4. Drizzle with melted chocolate, if needed, and freeze again until chocolate is solid then individually wrap ice cream sandwiches in plastic wrap. Freeze for up to 1 week. Let them soften outside of the freezer for a couple of minutes before serving.

NUTRITION

Calories: 252 kcal | Carbohydrates: 31g | Protein: 7g | Fat: 14g | Saturated Fat: 1g | Cholesterol: 53 mg | Sodium: 364 mg | Potassium: 20mg | Fiber: 3g | Sugar: 7g | Vitamin A: 75IU | Vitamin C: 1mg | Calcium: 28mg | Iron: 1.4mg

Baked Vegan Carrot Hash Browns

Servings size: 4 Prep Time: 15 mins

INGREDIENTS
- 2 cups grated carrots

- 1/2 cup coarsely chopped green scallions (green parts only for low FODMAP)
- 1/2 cup gluten-free flour
- 2 tablespoons ground flaxseeds
- 1 teaspoon ground cumin
- 1/2 teaspoon paprika
- Salt and pepper to taste
- 3-4 tablespoons olive oil

INSTRUCTIONS

1. Preheat the oven to 375°F (190°C) and line a baking sheet with parchment paper.
2. In a large bowl, add the grated carrots, green scallions, gluten-free flour, ground flaxseeds, cumin, paprika, salt, and pepper.
3. Form the mixture into tiny patties and set them on the prepared baking sheet.
4. Drizzle the patties with olive oil.
5. Bake for 25-30 minutes, or until the hash browns are golden brown and crispy.
6. Serve hot and enjoy!

NUTRITION

Calories: 160, Total Fat: 8g, Saturated Fat: 1g,, Cholesterol: 0mg, Sodium: 120mg, Total Carbohydrates: 20g, Dietary Fiber: 4g, Sugars: 4g Protein: 3g

---

Matcha Oats Low Fodmap

Makes: 1 Servings Prep Time: 5 minutes

INGREDIENTS

- 1/2 cup gluten-free rolled oats
- 1 tbsp chia seeds
- 1 teaspoon matcha powder
- 1/2 cup lactose-free milk or almond milk
- 1 tablespoon maple syrup (optional, adjust to taste)
- 1/4 teaspoon vanilla extract
- A pinch of salt
- Toppings (optional): sliced strawberries or banana, toasted coconut flakes, or low FODMAP almonds

INSTRUCTIONS

1. In a mason jar or airtight container, add oats, chia seeds, and matcha powder.
2. Pour in the lactose-free milk, maple syrup (if using), vanilla essence, and a sprinkle of salt. Stir well to mix.
3. Seal the container and refrigerate it overnight, or for at least 4 hours.
4. In the morning, give the mixture a toss and add your choice toppings before serving.

NUTRITION

Calories: 300, Carbohydrates: 45g, Protein: 8g, Fat: 10g, Fiber: 9g
Sugar: 10g, Sodium: 200mg

SNACKS RECIPES

Hummingbird Snack Cake with Low FODMAP

Serving size: 24   Prep Time: 10 mins
Total Time: 15 Mins

INGREDIENTS

- 2 /4 cups (399 g) plus 2 tablespoons low FODMAP
- gluten-free all-purpose flour, such as Bob's Red Mill, 2 3/4 cups (399 g) of wheat Gluten Free 1:1 Baking Flour to Flour
- 1.25 cups (or 218 grammes) of sugar
- The baking soda, one teaspoon:
- 100 milligrammes of cinnamon
- One milligramme of salt
- 1 cup (240 ml) vegetable oil, such as canola or rice bran
- 3 big eggs, at room temperature
- 2 medium sized ripe bananas, chopped into 1/2-inch (12 mm) rounds

- 1 cup (100 g) toasted pecan halves, chopped
  1 cup (225 g) canned crushed pineapple, gently drained
- 1 1/2 tablespoons vanilla extract
- Confectioners' Sugar, optional
- 1 recipe Lactose-Free Cream Cheese Frosting, optional

INSTRUCTIONS

1. Preheat the oven to 350°F/180°C. Coat the interior of a 13 x 9-inch (33 cm x 23 cm) pan with nonstick spray. Dust gently with more flour, shaking off excess.
2. Whisk together flour, sugar, baking soda, cinnamon and salt in a large basin to blend and aerate; put aside.
3. In a separate medium-sized bowl, mix together the oil and eggs until thoroughly incorporated. Stir in bananas, nuts, pineapple and vanilla.
4. Pour wet ingredients over dry and mix until incorporated. Batter will be heavy; make sure you mix completely and there are no pockets of flour remaining. Scrape into the prepared pan and smooth top with a tiny offset spatula.

5. Bake for approximately 35 to 40 minutes or until a wooden skewer reveals a few moist crumbs. Cool pan on rack until totally cooled. Cake is ready to frost - or serve as is, or sprinkled lightly with confectioners' sugar.

6. If using frosting, make sure it is smooth and creamy and spreadable. Cover the whole cake top with casual swirls of frosting, using an icing spatula or even the back of a spoon. Cake may be served immediately or refrigerated at cool room temperature in a sealed container for up to 3 days.

NUTRITION

Calories: 253 kcal | Carbohydrates: 33g | Protein: 3g | Fat: 13g | Saturated Fat: 1g | Sodium: 150mg | Fiber: 1g | Sugar: 17g | Calcium: 1mg

---

Low Fodmap Chocolate Cake

Serving size: 24 Prep Time: 10 mins
Cook Time: 35 mins. Total Time: 45 mins

INGREDIENTS

- 2 ¾ cups (399 g) low FODMAP gluten-free all-purpose flour, such as Bob's Red Mill 1:1 Baking Flour to Flour
- 2 cups (396 g) sugar
- ⅔ cup (56 g) Scattered natural cocoa
- 2 tablespoons baking soda
- One milligramme of salt
- 2 cups (480 ml) room-temperature water
- ⅔ cup (165 ml) neutral vegetable oil, such as canola, rice bran or sunflower
- 2 tablespoons apple cider or distilled white vinegar
- 1 tablespoon vanilla extract

INSTRUCTIONS

1. Position a rack in the middle of your oven. Preheat the oven to 350°F (180°C). Coat two 8- or 9-inch (20 or 23 cm) round cake pans with nonstick spray, cover the bottoms with parchment circles, then spray the paper. (see Tips below if using the recommended alternate pans).
2. Whisk together flour, sugar, cocoa, baking soda and salt in a large basin.

3. Whisk together water, oil, vinegar and vanilla in a medium basin.

4. Pour wet over dry and whisk until mixed and smooth. Divide batter equally in prepared pans. Firmly tap the bottom of the pan on the work surface to remove any bubbles.

5. Bake for approximately 25 to 35 minutes or until a toothpick reveals a few moist crumbs. Cool pan on rack for 15 minutes. Unmold the cake onto a rack, take off paper and cool fully. Cake is ready to fill and frost. Alternatively, put a layer on cardboard round and double wrap in plastic wrap; keep at room temperature and assemble within 24 hours, which is my choice. You may also triple wrap and freeze for up to 1 month. Defrost in the refrigerator overnight.

NUTRITION

Calories: 196 kcal | Carbohydrates: 35g | Protein: 1g | Fat: 6g | Sodium: 188mg | Fiber: 1g | Sugar: 20g

Low Fodmap Sour Cream Apple Streusel Cake

Serving size: 24   Prep Time: 15 minutes
Cook Time: 40 mins Total Time: 55 mins

INGREDIENT

Streusel:

- 3/4 cup (75 g) pecan halves chopped ¾ cup (160 g) tightly packed light brown sugar
- 3 tablespoons melted unsalted butter
- 2 tablespoons low FODMAP gluten-free all-purpose flour, such as Bob's Red Mill 1:1 Baking Flour to Flour
- 1 ½ teaspoons cinnamon

Cake:

- 1 3/4 cups (254 g) low FODMAP gluten-free all-purpose flour, such as Bob's Red Mill 1:1 Baking Flour to Flour
- 1 teaspoon baking powder; use gluten-free if following a gluten-free diet
- The baking soda, one teaspoon:
- 1/4 teaspoon salt
- 1/2 cup (113 g; 1 stick) unsalted butter, at room temperature, cut into pieces
- 1 cup (198 g) sugar

- 1 teaspoon vanilla extract
- 2 big eggs, at room temperature
- 1 cup (240 g) lactose-free sour cream, at room temperature
- 280 g (2 cups) diced peeled apples, such as Pink Lady

INTRODUCTION:

1. Preheat the oven to 350°F (180°C). Coat a 13 x 9-inch (33 cm x 23 cm) pan with nonstick spray.
2. For the Streusel: Combine all of the streusel ingredients together in a small bowl until equally blended; put aside.

For the Cake:

1. Whisk together the flour, baking powder, baking soda, and salt in a small dish to aerate and combine; leave aside.
2. In the bowl of a stand mixer equipped with the paddle attachment, beat the butter on medium-high speed until creamy, approximately 2 minutes. Gradually add the sugar and continue to beat on medium-high speed until extremely light and fluffy, approximately 3 minutes. Beat in the vanilla extract. (You can do this with a hand-held

71

electric mixer, but beating times will be longer; utilize visual signals).

3. Add the eggs one at a time, beating thoroughly after each addition. Add the flour mixture in three batches alternating with sour cream, starting and finishing with the flour mixture. When a few floury streaks still remain, mix in the apples until flour is fully integrated.

4. Scrape batter into prepared pan and smooth the top. Scatter streusel evenly over the top. Bake until a bamboo skewer inserted into the cake shows a few moist crumbs adhering when withdrawn, approximately 30 to 40 minutes. Cool in the pan on a rack. The cake is ready to serve. Cut into a 6 x 4 grid to produce the 24 serving size pieces of cake. Cake may be kept at room temperature for up to three days wrapped properly with plastic wrap and aluminum foil (I use both).

NUTRITION

Calories: 190 kcal | Carbohydrates: 26g | Protein: 2g | Fat: 9g | Sodium: 83mg | Fiber: 0.5g | Sugar: 16g

Low Fodmap Cake Bliss Balls

Serving size: 12 Prep Time: ten mins
Total Time: 10 mins

INGREDIENTS

- 1 cup (99 g) old-fashioned oats; use gluten-free if following a gluten-free diet
- 1/2 cup (135 g) natural peanut butter
- 1/3 cup (75 ml) maple syrup
- 1 tablespoon ground flaxseed
- 1 teaspoon vanilla extract
- ¼ cup (48 g) multi-colored sprinkles, plus additional if desired

INSTRUCTIONS

1. Place oats, PB, maple syrup, flaxseeds and vanilla essence in a bowl and whisk together very well with a strong wooden spoon, big, firm silicone spatula or your hands until fully blended. We prefer to use our stand mixer equipped with the flat paddle and definitely suggest this strategy. Once the mixture is fully and evenly blended, fold in the colored sprinkles.

2. Roll the mixture into tiny, bite-size balls approximately 1-inch (2.5 cm) across. We use a little scoop to facilitate the procedure. If the mixture is too soft, just cover with plastic wrap and chill until stiff enough to roll. If you prefer, you may add a few more sprinkles to the exterior of the balls as well as shown. Refrigerate in an airtight container for up to 1 week or freeze up to 1 month.

NUTRITION

Calories: 180 kcal | Carbohydrates: 23g | Protein: 5g | Fat: 8g | Saturated Fat: 1g | Sodium: 2mg | Potassium: 91mg | Fiber: 3g | Sugar: 7g | Calcium: 19mg | Iron: 0.9mg

---

Toasted Marshmallow Chocolate Crispy Snacks

Serving size: 25 Prep Time: 20 mins
Cook Time: 5 mins Total Time: 25 mins

INGREDIENTS

- 6 cups (240 g) Envirokidz Choco Chimps Cereal

- 4 tablespoons unsalted butter, sliced into pieces
- 6 cups (270 g) little marshmallows

INSTRUCTIONS

1. Preheat broiler with rack positioned pretty near to the heat source.
2. Coat a big, wide heatproof bowl with nonstick spray; add cereal in the bowl. Coat a big silicone spatula with nonstick spray as well. Line an 8-inch square pan with plastic wrap and coat with nonstick spray and put all of them aside.
3. Scatter butter evenly over a rimmed half-sheet pan. Scatter marshmallows evenly all over the pan. Place under the broiler and observe attentively. In less than 3 minutes the marshmallows should melt, bubble up and begin to color. Use the time cues as a recommendation. You want the marshmallows to be thoroughly browned but not burnt. Using hot gloves gently take the skillet from the oven and tilt it over the dish of cereal. Use the silicone spatula to scrape butter/marshmallow mixture over the cereal

and fold everything together until fully incorporated.

4. Scrape into a prepared pan (let to cool slightly if required) and use moist fingertips and palms to press down into an equal coating. Allow it to sit until solid and set, approximately an hour, or speed this process by refrigerating quickly (about 15 minutes).

5. Pull up on plastic wrap and remove the solid square from the pan. Set on the work surface and peel plastic away and cut into a 5 by 5 grid into 25 bars. These are best served the same day but may be refrigerated in an airtight container at room temperature for up to 3 days.

6. Coat a big silicone spatula with nonstick spray and leave aside. Line an 8-inch (20 cm) square pan with plastic wrap and cover with nonstick spray; put aside.

7. Melt butter in a large saucepan over medium heat. Add marshmallows and melt over medium heat, stirring often. When marshmallows are roughly three-quarters melted add the espresso powder and cinnamon and mix aggressively until

marshmallows are totally melted and espresso dissolved. Turn heat off and immediately add cereal to melted marshmallow mixture and use coated spatula to fold together and blend thoroughly. Scrape mixture into prepared pan (let cool momentarily if too hot) and use moist fingertips and palms to push down into an equal layer. Allow it to sit until solid and set, approximately an hour, or speed this process by refrigerating quickly (about 15 minutes).

8. Pull up on plastic wrap and remove from the pan. Set on the work surface and pull the plastic away. Cut the 5 by 5 grid into 25 bars. These are great if served the same day but they may be kept in an airtight container at room temperature for up to 3 days.

NUTRITION

Calories: 232 kcal | Carbohydrates: 54g | Protein: 1g | Fat: 2g | Saturated Fat: 1g | Sodium: 45mg | Potassium: 3mg | Fiber: 1g | Sugar: 36g | Calcium: 2mg | Iron: 0.1mg

Keto Deviled Eggs

Serving size 12 Total time: 25 mins

INGREDIENTS

- 12 eggs that have been cooked and allowed to cool, hard-boiled
- 1 tablespoon of mustard labeled Dijon
- 1.5 milligrammes of spicy sauce
- half a cup of mayonnaise
- 2 tablespoons of vinegar made from white wine
- Paprika, to be used as a topping, one teaspoon per serving

INSTRUCTIONS

1. Peel your hard-boiled eggs and slice each one in half lengthwise.
2. Use your hands or a spoon to remove the cooked yolk from each egg.
3. Set the empty egg halves on a serving dish.
4. Place the egg yolks in a medium mixing dish and use a fork to crush the egg yolks.
5. Then, add the mustard, spicy sauce, mayonnaise, and vinegar to the bowl. Use a

spatula to mix together the ingredients until smooth.

6. Place the egg yolk mixture into the bottom corner of a big plastic zip-top bag (or a piping bag). Cut the corner off the bottom of the bag with scissors and then gently pipe the egg yolk mixture into each of the empty egg halves.

7. Sprinkle the tops of the deviled eggs with paprika and serve refrigerated or at room temperature.

NUTRITION

Calories: 115 Sugar: 0.3 gSodium: 150.2 mgFat: 9.3 gSaturated Fat: 2.3 gCarbohydrates: 0.5 gFiber: 0 gProtein: 6.3 gCholesterol: 188.6 mg

---

Low FODMAP Snack Bars with Protein & Fiber

Servings size 12   Prep Time: 15 mins
Cook Time: 5 mins Chilling Time: 30 mins
Total Time: 50 minutes

INGREDIENTS

- 1 cup (256 g) no-stir type chunky peanut butter, such as Skippy
- ½ cup (120 ml) unsweetened almond milk
- 1/3 cup (75 ml) maple syrup
- 2 cups (198 g) rolled oats; use gluten-free if following a gluten-free diet
- 1 cup (120 g) FODMAP Foods Vanilla Gut Friendly Protein Meal Replacement Shake powder
- ¼ cup (56 g) tiny semisweet chocolate chips; use vegan if following a vegan diet
- ¼ cup (42 g) raisins
- 1 teaspoon cinnamon

INSTRUCTIONS

1. Coat the interior of an 8-inch (20 cm) square pan with nonstick spray. (If you use a pan with square edges, you will obtain nicer looking bars in the end).

2. Place peanut butter, almond milk, and maple syrup in a medium size pot. Heat over low-medium heat, whisking periodically, just until the mixture feels warm, which will only take a few minutes. Whisk the items together so that they are incorporated thoroughly.

3. Remove from heat and mix in the oats, meal replacement powder, chocolate chips, raisins, and cinnamon. The warmth of the mixture will melt the chocolate chips, which is what you want. As they stiffen up, they will assist the bars hold together.

4. Spread the mixture into the pan, using a silicone spatula to produce an equal surface. Chill the bars in the pan until stiff enough to cut, approximately 30 minutes. You may also simply leave at room temperature for a few hours. The time is not as crucial as the stiffness in texture. Cut into a 3 by 4 grid to yield 12 bars. Bars are ready to serve. You may keep at room temperature in an airtight container for up to 4 days or freeze in an airtight container for up to a month. They thaw rapidly.

NUTRITION

Calories: 277 kcal | Carbohydrates: 29g | Protein: 11g | Fat: 14g | Saturated Fat: 0.01g | Polyunsaturated Fat: 0.01g | Monounsaturated Fat: 0.001g | Sodium: 2mg | Potassium: 55mg | Fiber: 3g | Sugar: 6g | Vitamin C: 0.3mg | Calcium: 9 mg | Iron: 0.1mg

Low FODMAP Chewy Granola Bars

Serving size: 16 Prep Time: 10 mins
Cook Time: 30 mins Total Time: 40 mins

INGREDIENTS

- 1 2/3 cups (164 g) old-fashioned oats (use gluten-free if on a gluten-free diet)
- 1/2 cup (80 g) dried cranberries
- 1/2 cup (83 g) raisins
- 1/2 cup (54 g) toasted pecan or walnut halves, chopped
- 1/3 cup (32 g) almond flour, produced from blanched or natural almonds
- 1/4 cup (17 g) unsweetened shredded coconut
- 1/4 cup (35 g) sunflower seeds
- 1/2 teaspoon cinnamon
- 1/2 teaspoon salt
- 1/3 cup (75 ml) creamy, smooth peanut butter (see Tips)
- 1/3 cup (66 g) sugar
- 1/3 cup (75 ml) vegetable oil, such as canola or safflower
- 1/4 cup (60 ml) maple syrup

- 2 teaspoons rice malt syrup
- 1 tablespoon water
- 1 teaspoon vanilla essence

INSTRUCTIONS

1. Position rack in center of oven. Preheat the oven to 350°F/180°C. Line an 8-inch (20 cm) square pan with aluminum foil or parchment and coat foil or paper with nonstick spray.

2. Place oats, cranberries, raisins, nuts, almond flour, coconut, sunflower seeds, cinnamon and salt in the bowl of a stand mixer equipped with a flat paddle and blend until incorporated on low speed. Alternately you may mix together by hand in a big basin.

3. Whisk together the peanut butter, sugar, oil, maple syrup, rice malt syrup, water and vanilla in a small bowl until incorporated and smooth. Add to the dry mix and blend until everything is equally combined. A mixer makes this simple; if preparing by hand it will require a little elbow grease, but it can be done! Use a mix of a wooden spoon and silicone spatula if making by hand.

4. Scrape mixture into prepared pan leveling and smoothing the surface with a little offset spatula.

5. Bake for approximately 30 minutes or until a toothpick inserted in the middle tests clean. Cool pan on rack. Lift foil or paper out of the pan, peel away, and cut into a 4 × 4 grid to make 16 bars. The bars may be kept in an airtight container at room temperature for up to 3 days. Or, do what we do and wrap bars individually with plastic wrap, throw all of them in a zip top bag and keep in the freezer for up to a month. This makes it extremely simple to grab on one-the-go and they thaw quite rapidly.

NUTRITION

Calories: 327 kcal | Carbohydrates: 41g | Protein: 6g | Fat: 16g | Saturated Fat: 2g | Sodium: 80mg | Potassium: 205mg | Fiber: 5g | Sugar: 14g | Vitamin C: 0.5mg | Calcium: 25mg | Iron: 1.6mg

---

Low Fodmap Chex Mix Snack

Servings size 24 Prep Time: 5 mins

Cook Time: 45 mins   Total Time: 50 mins

INGREDIENTS

- 1 1/2 tbsp unsalted butter
- 1 1/2 teaspoons Garlic-Infused Oil, prepared using either vegetable or olive oil, or bought equivalent
- 2 teaspoons Worcestershire sauce
- 1/2 teaspoon salt
- 1/8 teaspoon cayenne, optional
- 3 cups (90 g) Rice Chex
- 1/2 cup (70 g) total combination of peanuts, almonds, macadamias, and pecans
- 1/2 cup tiny gluten-free pretzels

INSTRUCTIONS

1. Position rack in center of oven. Preheat the oven to 250°F/121°C. Have a rimmed half-sheet pan nearby.
2. Melt the butter and oil together in a big microwave safe bowl. Whisk in Worcestershire sauce, salt and cayenne, if using. Fold in cereal, nuts and pretzels until uniformly covered. It will be a light covering. Scrape Chex Mix out onto a rimmed sheet pan.

3. Bake for approximately 30 to 45 minutes or until gently brown, rotating once throughout baking. Cool pan on rack. Chex Mix is ready to consume or may be kept in an airtight container for up to 1 week at cool room temperature

NUTRITION

Calories: 138 kcal | Carbohydrates: 26g | Protein: 2g | Fat: 3g | Saturated Fat: 1g | Sodium: 319 mg | Potassium: 53mg | Fiber: 1g | Sugar: 2g | Vitamin A: 550IU | Vitamin C: 6.6mg | Calcium: 110mg | Iron: 9.9mg

---

Roasted Chickpeas

Servings size: 12 Prep Time: 30 mins
Cook Time: 35 mins Total Time: 1 hour 5 mins

INGREDIENTS
- 2, 15.5-ounce (439 g) cans chickpeas
- washed and drained 3 tablespoons oil either vegetable oil, extra virgin olive oil, coconut oil or Garlic-Infused Oil

INSTRUCTIONS

1. Drain the chickpeas in a strainer, give them a short rinse under cold water, then pour them in a big bowl and cover with cool water. Use your hands to press the chickpeas together gently under the water to release the outer skins, which will float to the top. You may not get them all, which is good, but attempt to eliminate most of them. Skim off the skins and toss them away then drain the chickpeas thoroughly again.

2.

3. Lay a huge number of triple layered paper towels on your counter and pour the chickpeas on top. Cover with extra paper towels and gently but completely pat them as dry as possible. Some additional skins could fall free; trash them.

4. Now, this following step is an optional step; it all depends on how big of a hurry you are in. I prefer to put the towel-dried chickpeas out on a rimmed sheet pan and allow them to air dry for 30 minutes. I believe this additional drying phase helps them crisp up in the oven more uniformly. But, you may also simply move to the next stage straight away if you

choose. Meanwhile, Position rack in the center of the oven. Preheat the oven to 400°F/200°C.

5.

6. Dump the chickpeas in a bowl, add oil of choice and fold to coat thoroughly and evenly.

7.

8. Now sprinkle the dry chickpeas on the rimmed sheet pan, equally spaced. Roast for 15 minutes, then shake pan to rotate the chickpeas, then roast for approximately 15 more minutes or until they are golden brown, dry and crisp. You could need a few more minutes; go by texture, not time!

9. As soon as you take the Roasted Chickpeas from the oven, continue to flavor them as you want or come up with your own low FODMAP ideas. Allow them to cool, then store in sealed containers for up to 4 days. They could survive longer, depending on how effective you were at drying them out.

NUTRITION

Calories: 47 kcal | Carbohydrates: 1g | Protein: 1g | Fat: 5g | Saturated Fat: 1g | Sodium: 1mg | Sugar: 1g

Low Fodmap Mocha Espresso Power Balls

Serving size 12 Prep Time: 10 mins
Total Time: 10 minutes

INGREDIENTS

- 1 cup (99g) old-fashioned oats; substitute gluten-free if following a gluten-free diet
- 1/2 cup (135 g) no-stir style creamy peanut butter; I utilize Skippy
- 1/3 cup (75 ml) rice syrup
- 1 tablespoon + 1 teaspoon Dutch-processed cocoa
- 2 tablespoons instant powdered espresso
- 1/8 teaspoon vanilla extract
- ¼ cup (44 g) chocolate covered espresso beans, crushed

INSTRUCTIONS

1. Place oats, peanut butter, rice syrup, cocoa, espresso and vanilla in a bowl and mix together very well with a strong wooden spoon, big, firm silicone spatula or your

hands until well blended. We prefer to use our stand mixer equipped with the flat paddle and definitely suggest this strategy. Once the mixture is fully and evenly blended, fold in the crushed chocolate coated espresso beans.

2. Roll the mixture into tiny, bite-size balls approximately 1-inch (2.5 across. I use a little scoop to facilitate the procedure. If the mixture is too soft, just cover with plastic wrap and chill until stiff enough to roll. Refrigerate in an airtight container for up to 1 week or freeze up to 1 month.

NUTRITION

Calories: 174 kcal | Carbohydrates: 22g | Protein: 6g | Fat: 8g | Saturated Fat: 1g | Sodium: 6mg | Potassium: 78mg | Fiber: 3g | Sugar: 6g | Calcium: 15mg | Iron: 0.9mg

---

Low Fodmap Sweet Spicy Kettle Corn

Servings size: 12 Prep Time: 5 mins
Cook Time: 10 mins   Total Time: 15 mins

INGREDIENTS

- 1/4 cup (60 ml) neutral vegetable oil, such as canola or rice bran oil
- 2/3 cup (140 g) popcorn kernels, ideally organic
- 1/3 cup (65 g) sugar (white or firmly packed light brown sugar (71 g))
- 1 teaspoon kosher salt
- 1/2 teaspoon cinnamon
- 1/4 teaspoon chipotle pepper or to taste

INSTRUCTIONS

1. Place ¼ cup (60 ml) vegetable oil in a large (at least 6-quart/5.7 L) covered saucepan. Add a few corn kernels, cover and cook over low heat. When you hear the kernels burst, add the remaining kernels and sugar, cover, and continue to simmer, stirring the pot often. Do not walk away! Listen to the popping noises and when they calm down, vent the lid to enable steam to escape.
2. With kettle corn I do not wait until all the popping noises end; I actually take the pot from the heat while there is still a little popping activity; this will reduce burning from the caramelization of the sugar.

3. Pour popped corn into a large serving basin. Sprinkle it with salt, cinnamon and chipotle pepper and mix thoroughly. Sweet n' Spicy Kettle Corn is ready to serve and we appreciate it best consumed as soon as possible. It can keep for a few days in an airtight container held at room temperature (or even up to a week), but there is nothing like having this extremely fresh!

NUTRITION

Calories: 110 kcal | Carbohydrates: 16g | Protein: 1g | Fat: 5g | Saturated Fat: 1g | Sodium: 194mg | Fiber: 1g | Sugar: 7g

LUNCH & DINNER

Low Fodmap Salmon Salade Nicoise

Servings size: 8   Prep Time: 30 minutes
Cook Time: 20 mins Total Time: 50 mins

INGREDIENTS

- 8- ounces (225 g) little thin-skinned potatoes, such as purple, red or fingerling potatoes
- Kosher salt
- 4- ounces (115 g) slender green beans, ideally haricots verts, trimmed
- 6 big eggs, room temperature
- 2 tablespoons extra virgin olive oil
- ¼ cup (32 g) drained brined capers, patted dry
- 1- pound (455 g) skin-on salmon filet
- Freshly ground black pepper
- 4 flat anchovy filets wrapped in oil
- ½ cup (120 ml) Low FODMAP Lemon Salad Dressing, prepared with coarse ground mustard
- 4 cups (500 g) shredded frisée

- 12 slices of watermelon radish 8 cherry or grape tomatoes, whole or halved ¼ cup (30 g) pitted Niçoise olives

INSTRUCTIONS

1. Place potatoes in a medium sized saucepan and add cold water to adequately cover; salt the water. Bring to a boil, lower heat to a vigorous simmer, and cook until knife-tender, approximately 15-minutes. Transfer potatoes to a half-sheet pan using a slotted spoon.
2. Return the same saucepan and water to a boil and cook the green beans until crisp-tender, approximately 2 minutes. Using a slotted spoon to transfer to a bowl of icy water. Chill until cold, then drain and pat dry.
3. Return water in the saucepan to a boil again and cook the eggs for 8 minutes. Transfer eggs to a basin of ice water and chill until cold. Peel, then put aside.
4. Meanwhile, heat 2 tablespoons of the oil in a small saucepan over medium-high. Add capers and heat, rotating pan regularly, until capers burst, but take care not to let them burn and blacken. Transfer capers with a

slotted spoon to paper towels to drain; set aside.

5. Preheat the oven to 425°F (220°C). Place salmon skin side down on a half-sheet pan. Brush with remaining caper oil and season with salt and pepper. Roast until medium-rare — salmon should be slightly transparent in the middle – approximately 10 to 12 minutes. Cool to room temperature.

6. Meanwhile, in a small bowl, mash the anchovies with a fork, then stir in Lemon Salad Dressing. Taste and season with salt and pepper.

To Serve:

- Arrange frisée on a dish, sprinkle with a little dressing and toss to coat. Break salmon into big flaky pieces using a fork or your fingers, removing it from the skin, which you can discard (or give it to your dog as I do). Arrange on frisée. Halve the potatoes and peeled eggs and put on a tray along with green beans and radishes. Scatter tomatoes and olives around and top with fried capers. Drizzle additional dressing over top and serve immediately.

NUTRITION

Calories: 264 kcal | Carbohydrates: 9g | Protein: 17g | Fat: 15g | Sodium: 119mg | Fiber: 1g | Sugar: 1g

---

Moroccan Lamb Shanks With Pomegranate & Mint

Makes: 4 servings   Prep Time: 10 mins
Cook Time: 50 mins   Total Time: 1 hour 30 mins

INGREDIENTS

- 1 teaspoon coriander seeds
- 1/2 teaspoon cumin seeds
- 1/2 teaspoon fennel seeds
- 1/4 teaspoon chili powder, ground red serrano chillis
- Kosher salt
- Freshly ground black pepper
- 4 (approximately 2 ½ pounds (1.2 kg)) lamb shanks, use New Zealand lamb for the smaller size
- 1 1/2 teaspoons cornstarch
- 2 tablespoons olive oil, virgin or extra virgin, divided 2 medium carrots, peeled and chopped into 2-inch chunks

- 1 cup (60 g) coarsely sliced leeks, green portions only
- 8 single sprigs thyme each around 3 to 4-inches (7.5 cm to 10 cm) long
- 1 cinnamon stick
- 1 1/2 cups (360 ml) unsweetened cranberry juice
- 1 1/2 cups (360 ml) water or low FODMAP Chicken Stock
- 1/4 cup (38 g) pomegranate seeds
- 1/4 cup (10 g) mint leaves

INSTRUCTIONS

1. Position rack in center of oven. Preheat oven to 350°/180°

2. Place coriander seeds, cumin seeds, fennel seeds, chili powder and 1 teaspoon salt in a strong zipper top plastic bag. Expel air and leave the bag open just a bit. Use a mallet to crush the spices straight through the bag or use a rolling pin. Aim for a coarsely ground texture.

3. Place shanks in a large basin and sprinkle with spice mixture and coat with several grinds of black pepper. Use your hands to run it in as evenly as possible. Let rest for 30

minutes or cover and chill overnight. Bring back to room temperature, if chilly. Sprinkle cornstarch over lamb and again use fingers to massage it over the meat in a uniform layer.

4. Heat 1 tablespoon of oil in a large straight-sided pan or Dutch oven over medium heat until it shimmers. Add shanks and heat until browned on both sides, approximately 10 minutes total. Use tongs to turn them around.

5. Once they are browned, move them to a plate. Add remaining 1 tablespoon oil to the skillet still over medium heat and add carrots and leeks. Use a wooden spatula to scrape up any browned parts from the bottom of the pan and cook, stirring once or twice, for approximately 2 minutes or until leeks begin to soften.

6. Add thyme, cinnamon stick, cranberry juice and water, mix to incorporate, and bring to a boil. Add shanks with any of the spice mixture that may have dropped off and season with salt and pepper.

7. Cover the pot and put it in the oven. Braise for 1 hour, then check liquid level, making

sure there is at least 1-inch (2.5 cm) of liquid in pot adding extra water if required

8. Continue braising for approximately 30 minutes longer, then test doneness. The flesh should be extremely soft and fall off the bone. The flesh will also have receded and the bones will be seen as shown in the picture.

9. Remove the thyme stems and cinnamon stick. The meal is ready to serve or chill, refrigerate in an airtight container and keep for up to 3 days. Reheat on the stovetop. Adjust spices if required and spread pomegranate seeds and mint leaves over the dish shortly before serving. We adore this paired with rice and a green salad.

NUTRITION

Calories: 738 kcal | Carbohydrates: 26g | Protein: 54g | Fat: 45g | Saturated Fat: 1g | Sodium: 13mg | Potassium: 200mg | Fiber: 4g | Sugar: 14g | Vitamin A: 765IU | Vitamin C: 17.7mg | Calcium: 69mg | Iron: 1.7mg

Low Fodmap Chili Mac

Servings size: Prep Time: 15 mins
Cook Time: 30 mins   Total Time: 45 mins

INGREDIENTS

- 8- ounces (225 g) low FODMAP gluten-free macaroni, such as Jovial
- 1 teaspoon Garlic-Infused Oil, prepared using vegetable oil
- 1 cup (64 g) freshly cut scallions, green parts only
- 1 green bell pepper, cored, diced
- 1- pound (455 g) lean ground beef, ideally at least 80% lean
- 2 tablespoon cumin
- ½ teaspoon dried oregano
- ½ teaspoon smoked paprika
- ¼ teaspoon cayenne
- ¼ teaspoon chipotle powder
- ½ teaspoon kosher salt, plus additional
- Freshly ground black pepper
- 1 cup (240 ml) low FODMAP Beef Stock
- 1 cup (242 g) canned chopped tomatoes, with juice
- 1 cup (250 g) canned tomato purée

- ½ cup (105 g) canned, drained black beans
- ½ cup (105 g) canned, drained pinto beans
- 3- ounces (85 g) sharp cheddar cheese, shredded
- 3- ounces (85 g) mozzarella, shredded

INSTRUCTIONS

1. Cook your macaroni in a big saucepan of salted boiling water until a bit harder than al dente, drain and put aside.
2. Heat the Garlic-Infused Oil in a large Dutch-oven over low heat and sauté the chopped scallion greens until starting to soften, then add the green pepper and sauté for another minute or two.
3. Add the ground beef, breaking it up thoroughly and cook over medium heat until it is approximately halfway cooked through, then add the cumin, oregano, paprika, cayenne, chipotle powder, ½ teaspoon salt and ample grindings of black pepper. Keep sautéing until the meat is no longer pink.
4. Add the beef stock, chopped tomatoes, tomato purée, black beans and pinto beans and whisk everything together thoroughly. Cover, adjust heat and simmer for

approximately 15 minutes to build flavor. Meanwhile, position the rack in the center of the oven and prepare the broiler to high. Taste the chili and adjust spice. Fold the macaroni into chili. Sprinkle the top with both cheeses and place under the broiler until the cheese is melted. Serve immediately. Leftovers may be refrigerated for up to 3 days and reheated in the microwave.

NUTRITION

Calories: 316 kcal | Carbohydrates: 32g | Protein: 23g | Fat: 11g | Saturated Fat: 3g | Cholesterol: 44mg | Sodium: 349 mg | Potassium: 231mg | Fiber: 2g | Sugar: 2g | Vitamin A: 197IU | Vitamin C: 1mg | Calcium: 73mg | Iron: 2mg

---

Low Fodmap Instant Pot Pork Ragu

Servings size 8 Prep Time: 15 minutes
Cook Time: 1 hour 30 mins   Total Time: 1 hour 45 mins

INGREDIENTS

- 1 ½ teaspoons Low FODMAP Garlic-Infused Oil, produced with olive oil
- 3- pound to 3 ½-pound (1.4 kg to 1.6 kg) bone-in or boneless pig butt or shoulder, at room temperature
- 3, 28- ounce (793 g) cans peeled plum tomatoes in purée
- ¾ cup (180 ml) Low FODMAP Chicken Stock or Low FODMAP Beef Stock ¾ cup (180 ml) dry red wine
- ¾ cup (48 g) freshly cut scallions, green parts only
- 1 medium trimmed and peeled carrot, coarsely chopped
- 1 medium trimmed stalk celery, finely, chopped
- 1 teaspoon kosher salt
- 1 teaspoon dried oregano
- 1 teaspoon dried rosemary
- ¾ teaspoon FreeFold Garlic Replacer ¾ teaspoon FreeFold Onion Replacer ¾ teaspoon freshly ground black pepper
- 3 tablespoons tomato paste
- Fresh flat-leaf parsley

INSTRUCTIONS

1. Press the Instant Pot button for Sauté and adjust the temperature to Medium/Normal/Custom 300°F (150°C). Set time for 10 minutes. Add the oil and let it heat up. Brown the meat in the oil on both sides.

2. Turn off the Sauté feature. Add the tomatoes and purée and smash the tomatoes a little with a potato masher or fork. Add the stock, wine, scallion greens, carrot, celery, salt, oregano, rosemary, Free Food Garlic Replacer, Free Food Onion Replacer and black pepper.

3. Lock the lid in place. Set the Instant Pot to Pressure Cook on Maximum for 1 hour with the Keep Warm option off. Press Start. Allow the pot to simmer and then restore to normal pressure on its own, which will take around 20 to 30 minutes after the allotted cooking period. Unlock the lid. Remove the pork to a big basin, where you may shred it with two forks.

4. Skim extra fat off of the surface of the sauce and discard. Set the machine to Sauté on Medium/Normal/Custom 300°F (150°C) for

20 minutes and hit Start. It will come to a simmer. Whisk in the tomato paste. Keep an eye on it, whisking regularly, and decrease it until it thickens a touch. Re-combine the sauce with the meat, stirring everything completely. Taste and adjust seasoning at this time. Your pork is ready to serve. We adore it with spaghetti, mashed potatoes or polenta. Serve a green salad on the side with a strong vinaigrette.

NUTRITION

Calories: 535 kcal | Carbohydrates: 18g | Protein: 30g | Fat: 35g | Saturated Fat: 1g | Polyunsaturated Fat: 1g | Monounsaturated Fat: 1g | Sodium: 338 mg | Potassium: 61mg | Fiber: 1g | Sugar: 1g | Vitamin A: 92IU | Vitamin C: 1mg | Calcium: 3mg | Iron: 1mg

---

Low FODMAP Baked Penne with Four Cheeses, Greens, and Tomatoes

Servings size: 8   Prep Time: 10 mins
Cook Time: 50 mins   Total Time: 1 hour

INGREDIENTS

- 1/4 cup 58 g + 1 tablespoon (½ stick plus 1 tablespoon) unsalted butter, softened, divided
- 2 cups (200 g) grated Parmigiano Reggiano cheese, split
- 1/4 cup (36 g) low FODMAP gluten-free all-purpose flour
- 4 cups (960 ml) lactose free whole milk, 2%, 1% or fat free at room temperature
- 3 ounces (85 g; roughly 1 cup) loosely packed coarsely shredded Havarti
- 1 big egg, at room temperature
- Kosher salt
- Freshly ground black pepper
- 1 pound (455 g) low FODMAP, gluten-free penne, such as rice based (cooked pasta weight is 910 g)
- 1 cup (20 g) fresh baby arugula or baby spinach leaves
- 1/2 cup (16 g) finely chopped fresh flat leaf parsley, divided 1 cup (210 g) lactose-free cottage cheese
- 5 3/4 ounces (160 g; roughly 2/3 cup) crumbled feta
- 3/4 dry pint (213 g) red or orange cherry or grape tomatoes, halved

INSTRUCTIONS:

1. Use the 1 tablespoon of butter to completely cover the bottom and insides of a 9-inch (23 cm) springform pan. Dust pan with ½ cup (50 g) of Parmigiano cheese all over.

2. Melt the remaining ¼ cup (58 g) of butter in a medium sized saucepan over medium heat. Whisk in flour to produce a roux and simmer for approximately 2 minutes to eliminate raw flavor, then gently whisk in milk. Bring to a boil, whisking constantly, and cook for approximately 10 minutes or until white sauce has thickened and displays whisk marks. Still overheat, add grated Havarti and 1 cup (100 g) Parmigiano and stir until melted and smooth. Whisk in egg and season with salt and pepper. Remove from heat and keep warm.

3. Position rack in middle of oven. Preheat oven to 375°F/190°

4. Bring a large saucepan with 5 quarts (4.7 L) of salted water to a boil and cook pasta until al dente; drain and add to a large mixing bowl. Add heated cheese sauce, baby greens or arugula and ¼ cup (8 g) parsley to

spaghetti and toss to incorporate. Stir in cottage cheese, feta and tomatoes. Pack mixture into prepared pan. Sprinkle reserved ½ cup (50 g) Parmigiano evenly on top.

5. Bake pasta for around 30 to 35 minutes or until the top is golden brown and a touch crusty. Let rest at least 20 minutes before unmolding. Sprinkle with reserved ¼ cup (8 g) parsley, cut into wedges and serve. Pasta may be served warm or at room temperature. Refrigerate leftovers well covered in plastic wrap and reheat in the microwave, if preferred.

NUTRITION

Calories: 574 kcal | Carbohydrates: 56g | Protein: 29g | Fat: 27g | Sodium: 449mg | Fiber: 3g | Sugar: 9g | Calcium: 4mg | Iron: 0.2mg

---

Low FODMAP Sesame Chicken

Servings size: 4   Prep Time 5 Mins
Cook Time 15 Mins   Total Time 20 Mins

INGREDIENTS

- 1/4 cup gluten-free all-purpose flour mix
- 1/4 teaspoon salt 1/4 teaspoon ground black pepper
- 1 1/2 pounds boneless, skinless chicken breasts (cut into thin strips across the grain)
- 2 tablespoons canola oil
- 1/4 cup reduced-sodium soy sauce or gluten-free tamari
- 1/4 cup granulated sugar
- 2 teaspoons toasted sesame seeds
- 1 teaspoon toasted sesame oil
- 1/4 cup fresh chopped chives

INSTRUCTIONS

1. In a large resealable plastic bag, mix the flour blend, salt and pepper. Add the chicken breast strips and shake well to coat.

2. Heat the canola oil in a large non-stick wok or pan over medium-high heat. Add the chicken and brown thoroughly, approximately 3 to 4 minutes a side.

3. Reduce heat to medium and transfer chicken to a platter and set aside. Add the soy sauce and sugar to the wok or pan and swirl and heat until sugar is dissolved. Stir in the

sesame seeds and sesame oil. Add the chicken back into the pan and toss lightly to coat. Remove from heat, mix in the chives and serve.

NUTRITION
Calories: 250-300, Protein: 15-20g,
Carbohydrates: 30-35g
Fat: 8-10g, Fiber: 5-7g

Low Fodmap Cilantro Lime Chicken

Servings size: 4 Total Time: 2 hours 25 mins

INGREDIENTS
- ½ bunch fresh cilantro (approximately ⅓ to ½ cup, chopped)
- ¼ cup fresh lime juice (approximately 2 limes)
- 2 teaspoons garlic-infused olive oil
- 2 tbsp extra-virgin olive oil
- 2 teaspoon packed brown sugar
- ½ teaspoon ground cumin
- ½ teaspoon kosher salt or sea salt

- 1 to 1.5 pounds boneless, skinless chicken breasts (approximately 2 big or 4 small)

INSTRUCTIONS

1. Place cilantro, lime juice, garlic-infused oil, olive oil, brown sugar, cumin, and salt in a blender. Blend until the cilantro is processed into little bits.
2. In a sealable container, insert chicken in the bottom. Pour cilantro lime marinade over the chicken and flip to coat. Refrigerate for at least 2 hours, but no more than 24 hours.
3. Cook chicken using your chosen method:

To broil or grill

- Preheat grill or broiler to 450°F or 500°F. Transfer the marinated chicken to the grill (or a broiler pan for the broiler) and discard any excess marinade. Grill (or broil) the chicken for 5 to 6 minutes each side, or until a food thermometer inserted into the thickest section registers 165°F. Let rest for 5 minutes. Slice and serve warm.

NUTRITION

Calories: 260, Total Fat: 11g
Saturated Fat: 2g, Cholesterol: 100mg

Sodium: 370mg, Total Carbohydrates: 4g
Dietary Fiber: 0g, Sugars: 2g, Protein: 35g

FODMAP Nourish Bowl

Prep Time: 10 mins. Cook Time. 20 mins
Total Time: 30 mins

INGREDIENTS

- 1/2 cup brown rice OR quinoa OR millet 3.5 ounces | 100g chicken breast OR tofu OR 1 egg
- 1.59 oz | 45g cherry tomatoes OR carrots OR spinach
- 1.41 oz | 40g canned chickpeas OR canned lentils OR sprouting mung beans 0.35 oz | 10g sunflower seeds OR sesame seeds OR pumpkin seeds

Dressing

- 3 tbsp olive oil extra virgin
- 1 tbsp apple cider vinegar OR lemon juice OR balsamic vinegar
- 1 tbsp mustard OR lactose free yogurt OR soy sauce
- Pinch of salt

- Pinch of black pepper

INSTRUCTIONS

1. Place your choice grain in 1 cup of boiling salted water. Reduce the heat to minimum and simmer for 20 minutes or until water evaporates and the grain is cooked. Fluff with a fork and put aside.

2. Choose one > EGG fry the egg in a pan with boiling water for 10 minutes | Chicken breast heat 2 tbsp of olive oil in a pan over medium–high heat. Add the chicken, sprinkle with salt and cook each side for 5 minutes or until meat is done | TOFU drain and wrap with a paper towel. Place a plate and a heavy item on top and leave aside for 10 minutes. Cut into squares and cover with salt and cumin. In a hot grill pan, cook for 5-10 minutes or until crispy and golden brown.

3. Choose one > cherry tomatoes cut in half | Carrots grate or ribbon with a potato peeler | Spinach heat 2 tbsp of olive oil in a skillet over medium–high heat. Add the spinach and sauté for 5 minutes or until spinach has wilted.

4. Drain and wash one of the pulses and put aside.

5. Assemble bowls in a lunch box. Cover the bottom with the grain. Add the protein, a vegetable and a pulse on top and sprinkle with the seeds. Place the cover and store in the fridge until eating.

6. For the dressing, in a small leak proof jar, mix all the ingredients and whisk until smooth. Place the cover and store in the fridge until eating.

7. You may enjoy the nourish bowl cold or gently heated in the microwave. Toss over the dressing before eating.

NUTRITION
Calories: 520, Total Fat: 32g, Saturated Fat: 5g
Cholesterol: 100mg, Sodium: 430mg
Total Carbohydrates: 38g, Dietary Fiber: 6g, Sugars: 3g, Protein: 23g

---

One Pot Low FODMAP Chicken and Rice

Servings size: 4 Prep Time: 15 mins
Cook Time: 35 mins Total Time: 50 mins

INGREDIENTS

- 4 skinless boneless chicken breasts, roughly 1 1/2 pounds
- 1/4 tablespoons sea salt
- 1/4 teaspoon black pepper
- 1 3/4 teaspoon ground cumin, divided
- 1 3/4 teaspoon paprika, split
- 1 tablespoon neutral flavored frying oil
- 1 red & green bell pepper, each, diced and deseeded*
- 1 big tomato, chopped
- 1 tablespoon ginger, chopped, fresh
- 1 teaspoon turmeric powder
- 1 cup white rice, uncooked
- 2 cups Casa De Santa Low FODMAP Vegetable Stock, prepare it by combining 2 teaspoons of the stock powder with 2 cups hot water
- 2 cups spinach

INSTRUCTIONS

1. Place the chicken breasts between two sheets of plastic cling wrap and pound them down to make them uniform in thickness. This will help the chicken cook evenly and produce

more tender chicken. Sprinkle each side of the chicken with salt, pepper, 1 teaspoon cumin and 1 teaspoon paprika.

2. Melt the oil in a big pan over a medium high heat on the stove. Add the chicken breasts and cook each side for 5-7 minutes or until browned on each side. Remove the chicken from a pan and place aside on a platter. The chicken doesn't need to be entirely cooked yet since you'll be returning it to the fire soon.

3. Add the chopped bell peppers, tomato, and ginger to the same pan and sauté for a few minutes to soften. Add the remaining 3/4 teaspoons of cumin and paprika along with the turmeric powder to the skillet. Mix the spices into the veggies to coat.

4. Stir in the uncooked rice and toss until the rice is covered with both spice and veggies. Pour the liquid into the pan and cover the rice. Carefully return the chicken back into the pan, cover with a fitting lid and simmer over a medium-low heat for 20 minutes until the liquid is nearly absorbed. Stir the spinach into the saucepan, cover and simmer until the liquid has all absorbed and the spinach is wilted.

5. Garnish with freshly cut cilantro and serve.

NUTRITION

Calories: 372 Saturated Fat: 4gCholesterol: 72mgSodium: 330mgCarbohydrates: 43gFiber: 2gSugar: 2gProtein: 30g

---

Low Fodmap Thai Curry Tofu & Green Beans

Servings size: 6   Prep Time: 10 mins
Cook Time: 15 mins   Total Time: 25 mins

INGREDIENTS

- 1, 14- ounce to 16-ounce (400 g to 455 g block) of extra-firm tofu
- 2 tablespoons ghee or Garlic-Infused Oil, produced with vegetable oil, or bought equivalent, divided ¼ cup (16 g) chopped scallions, green bits only
- 1 tablespoon Casa de Sante's Thai Curry Seasoning
- 2 medium beefsteak tomatoes, cored and chopped 8 ounces (225 g) fresh green beans, trimmed

- 1, 14.5 ounce (403 ml) can lite coconut milk or preferable 14-ounces UHT coconut milk, thoroughly mixed if canned
- Kosher salt
- Freshly ground black pepper
- Cilantro, optional

INSTRUCTIONS

1. Cut the tofu block in half lengthwise. arrange a triple layer of paper towel on a cutting board, arrange tofu slabs on top, then cover them with another triple layer of towel. Put something heavy on top, like another cutting board with a hefty pot on top. Allow to sit for approximately 10 minutes. This process will eliminate extra water from the tofu so that it will fry up with a wonderful crisp exterior texture.
2. Once tofu has drained, remove paper towels and cut tofu into cubes.
3. Heat a large, deep pan over medium heat and add 1 tablespoon of the ghee or oil (use oil for a vegan option) and cook until oil is shimmering. Add tofu and raise heat to medium-high. Cook undisturbed for a few minutes or until tofu is browned on the

bottoms, then toss around and continue to cook until well browned. Remove from pan and put aside, retaining heat.

4. Add remaining tablespoon of ghee or oil to the pan over medium heat.

5. Add scallions and sauté for approximately a minute or 2 until softened but not browned. Add Thai curry powder and mix around for 30 seconds, then add tomatoes and green beans and toss to coat, then coconut milk and whisk everything around together well. Adjust heat, partly cover and cook for approximately 3 minutes, then mix in tofu to coat with sauce and simmer for 5 more minutes or until heated through. Taste and season with salt and pepper as required. Your curry is ready to serve with or without a garnish of cilantro. And we enjoy this best with rice.

NUTRITION

Calories: 260 kcal | Carbohydrates: 8g | Protein: 9g | Fat: 23g | Fiber: 1g | Sugar: 1g

Coconut Tofu Curry

Serving size: 4   Prep Time: 10 mins
Cook Time: 15 mins. Total Time: 25 mins

INGREDIENTS

- 1, 14 to 16 -ounce (400 g to 455 g) block of extra-firm tofu 5 ounces (140 g) baby bok choy (these will be multiple little heads)
- 1 1/2 tablespoons + 2 teaspoons Garlic-Infused Oil prepared using vegetable oil, or bought equivalent, split
- 1/2 cup (32 g) sliced scallions, green parts only
- 1 tablespoon low FODMAP curry powder such as Frontier Co-op
- 1 tablespoon grated peeled fresh ginger
- 2 medium beefsteak tomatoes, cored and diced
- 3 medium carrots, peeled, stem end eliminated, sliced into big bite-size pieces on the diagonal
- 1, 14.5 ounce (403 ml) can lite coconut milk, thoroughly stirred
- 1/2 cup (15 g) fresh basil leaves, delicately torn

- 1 tablespoon fish sauce
- 1 tablespoon lime juice
- 1 tablespoon low-sodium soy sauce
- 2 teaspoons sugar

INSTRUCTIONS

1. Cut the tofu block in half lengthwise. arrange a triple layer of paper towel on a cutting board, arrange tofu slabs on top, then cover them with another triple layer of towel. Put something heavy on top, like another cutting board with a hefty pot on top. Allow to sit for approximately 10 minutes. This process will eliminate extra water from the tofu so that it will fry up with a wonderful crisp exterior texture.

2. While tofu is draining, prepare the young bok choy. Trim and discard the root ends. Dunk each young bok choy in a dish of lukewarm water and swirl it around to eliminate any debris. Dry completely, patting dry with a clean dish towel or paper towels. We normally leave the young bok choy intact but if they are on the large-ish side, cut lengthwise in half; put aside.

3. Once tofu has drained, remove paper towels and cut tofu into cubes.

4. Heat a large, deep pan over medium heat and add 1 ½ teaspoons oil and heat until oil is shimmering. Add tofu and raise heat to medium-high. Cook undisturbed for a few minutes or until tofu is browned on the bottoms, then toss around and continue to cook until well browned. Remove from pan and put aside, retaining heat.

5. Add remaining 2 tablespoons of oil with pan over medium heat. Add scallions and sauté for approximately a minute or 2 until softened but not browned. Add curry powder and ginger and stir around for 30 seconds, then add the bok choy, tomatoes, carrots, coconut milk, basil, fish sauce, lime juice, soy sauce and sugar and toss everything around together thoroughly. Adjust heat and cook for approximately 3 minutes, then toss in tofu to coat with sauce and simmer for 5 more minutes or until heated through. Coconut Tofu Curry is ready to serve. We prefer it with basmati rice.

NUTRITION

Calories: 268 kcal | Carbohydrates: 18g | Protein: 14g | Fat: 15g | Saturated Fat: 1g | Sodium: 524 mg | Potassium: 490 mg | Fiber: 5g | Sugar: 10g | Vitamin A: 4555 IU | Vitamin C: 45.7mg | Calcium: 108mg | Iron: 1.7mg

---

Penne Rigate With Gorgonzola, Radicchio & Walnuts

Serving size: 6 Prep Time: 10 mins
Cook Time: 12 mins Total Time: 22 mins

INGREDIENTS

- 1 cup (113 g) chopped walnuts
- Kosher salt
- 3/4 pound (340 g) gluten-free penne
- 1/4 cup (60 ml) olive oil
- 1 (approximately 1 pound; 455 g) head radicchio (ideally Treviso if you can locate it), cut into 1-inch-wide (2.5 cm) ribbons
- Freshly ground black pepper
- 6 ounces (170 g) crumbled Gorgonzola or other mild blue cheese

- 1/2 cup (16 g) chopped flat-leaf Italian parsley
- Orange zest, particularly from a blood orange; optional
- Grated Pecorino Romano cheese, for serving

INSTRUCTIONS

1. Heat a 12-inch (30.5 cm) skillet over medium heat. Add the walnuts and toast them over medium-low heat for approximately 4 minutes, stirring regularly so they do not burn. Remove and put aside. Wipe out the skillet.

2. Bring a big saucepan of water to a boil. Add 2 tablespoons of the salt and bring to a rolling boil. Add the pasta and boil until al dente according to package guidelines.

3. While the pasta boils, make the sauce: Heat the oil in a 12-inch (30.5 cm) skillet over medium-high heat. Add the radicchio and season with salt and pepper. Cook the radicchio until it starts to wilt and brown, approximately 5 minutes. Season with salt and pepper.

4. Stir in the Gorgonzola and simmer for 2 minutes. Add ½ cup (120 ml) of the pasta

water straight from the saucepan and boil for 3 minutes longer. The water should emulsify the cheese and give a silky texture.

5. Scoop the cooked pasta right into the pan and stir to incorporate the spaghetti with the sauce. Add the walnuts and parsley and toss again until glossy, adding ¼ cup (60 ml) of pasta water or more (up to 1 cup/240 ml), as required to soften up the sauce.

6. Plate in dishes and garnish with orange zest, if preferred. Season with salt and pepper and pass grated Pecorino Romano.

NUTRITION

Calories: 656 kcal | Carbohydrates: 50g | Protein: 18g | Fat: 46g | Saturated Fat: 4g | Sodium: 1mg | Potassium: 174mg | Fiber: 5g | Sugar: 1g | Vitamin C: 0.5mg | Calcium: 39mg | Iron: 1.2mg

---

Low Fodmap Sheet Pan Lasagna With Spicy Sausage & Spinach

Serving size: 8 Prep Time. 20 mins
Cook Time. 30 mins Total Time: 50 mins

INGREDIENTS

- Kosher salt
- 1- pound (455 g) low FODMAP, gluten-free lasagna noodles, such as Jovial brand, split into 2-inch (5 cm) pieces
- ¼ cup (60 ml) Garlic-Infused Oil, prepared from olive oil, handmade or bought, split
- 5- ounces (140 g) fresh baby spinach
- 1 cup (248 g) half skim or full-fat ricotta cheese; you may use lactose-free if make it, or can locate it
- Freshly ground pepper
- 1- pound (455 g) low FODMAP spicy Italian sausage, casings removed if required
- ¾ cup (48 g) sliced scallions, green parts only
- ¼ cup (28 g) minced leek bulb 4 cups (960 ml) low FODMAP marinara sauce, handmade or prepared
- 1/2 teaspoon red pepper flakes, optional
- 1- pound (455 g) shredded low moisture mozzarella, split
- 1 1/2 cups (125 g) freshly grated Parmesan, divided

INSTRUCTIONS

1. Preheat the oven to 425°F (220°C). Use 1 tablespoon of the oil to coat the interior of a commercial weight half-sheet pan, bottom and sides; leave aside.

2. Bring a big saucepan of salted water to a boil over high heat. Add lasagna pieces and cook, stirring constantly, until on the firm side of al dente. Remove ½ cup (120 ml) of the pasta water and save; drain the remaining pasta.

3. Meanwhile, heat 1 tablespoon of the oil in a large pan over medium heat. Add the spinach and simmer, turning constantly, until the spinach is nearly fully wilted. eliminate the spinach combination to a colander or strainer and press hard to eliminate any extra liquid; take time to properly dry up the spinach. Place the spinach in a medium-sized mixing bowl and use a pair of kitchen scissors to cut the spinach into bite-sized pieces. Add the ricotta cheese and whisk to mix. Season moderately with salt and liberally with pepper. Set aside.

4. Wipe out the skillet with paper towels and set over medium heat. Add the remaining 2 tablespoons of oil to the pan along with the

sausage and heat, tossing regularly and breaking apart as required, until the sausage is lightly browned, and cooked through, approximately 5 minutes. Add scallions and leek bulb to the pan and heat until the onion is aromatic and begins to soften, approximately another 3 minutes. Stir in marinara sauce, and optional red pepper flakes, if desired. Remove from the heat.

5. Stir in the pasta, pasta water, and approximately one-third of the mozzarella and Parmesan; you can do this by eye. Spread the spaghetti mixture over the prepared pan. Dollop the ricotta-spinach mixture here and there, then sprinkle with leftover mozzarella and Parmesan.

6. Bake until the pasta is soft, the sauce is bubbling, and the top is gently browned, approximately 30 minutes. Remove from the oven and allow rest for 5 minutes before serving. It can be a little sloppy looking on the plate, but believe us, no one ever complains.

NUTRITION

Calories: 730 kcal | Carbohydrates: 50g | Protein: 39g | Fat: 47g | Saturated Fat: 0.003g | Polyunsaturated Fat: 0.01g | Monounsaturated Fat: 0.004g | Sodium: 453mg | Potassium: 2mg | Fiber: 3g | Sugar: 4g | Vitamin A: 37IU | Vitamin C: 0.001mg | Calcium: 0.4mg | Iron: 0.02mg

---

Low Fodmap Pasta Primavera

Serving size: 6   Prep Time: 10 mins
Cook Time: 15 mins   Total Time: 25 mins

INGREDIENTS

- 2 tablespoons Onion-Infused Oil, produced with shallots and olive oil; additional if required
- 1/3 cup (24 g) chopped chives or scallion greens
- 3 1/2 cups (840 ml) water
- Kosher salt
- 12- ounces (340 g) low FODMAP, gluten-free penne, such as Jovial brand
- 3 asparagus stalks (50 g), trimmed, cut into 2-inch (5 cm) lengths

- 3- ounces (85 g) fresh baby arugula leaves
- 3- ounces (85 g) fresh baby spinach leaves
- 40 grams frozen peas, roughly ¼ cup
- 2 tablespoons unsalted butter
- 3- ounces (85 g) finely grated Parmesan cheese
- 2 tablespoons freshly squeezed lemon juice, plus 1 teaspoon finely grated lemon zest
- 2 teaspoons chopped fresh dill
- 2 teaspoons chopped fresh tarragon
- Freshly ground black pepper

INSTRUCTIONS

1. Heat the oil over medium heat in a big straight-sided skillet until shimmering (we used a pan 14-inch/35.5 cm wide and 3-inches/7.5 cm deep); you will need a cover for later. Add chives or scallion greens and sauté until tender, but not browned. Add the water, a big pinch of salt and the pasta, toss well, cover and bring to a boil. After 4 minutes add the asparagus and cook for approximately 30 seconds, then toss the arugula and spinach into the pasta and water. Re-cover the pot. Keep boiling until pasta is a bit stiffer than al dente. Do not allow the

water to entirely evaporate; the dish should seem juicy. Stir in the peas and leave it simmer for approximately 30 seconds, just to heat through.

2. Remove from heat; mix in butter, Parmesan, the lemon juice, zest, dill and tarragon. Toss everything together thoroughly; if the mixture seems dry, sprinkle in a bit of extra oil. Taste and season with salt and pepper and serve immediately.

NUTRITION

Calories: 325 kcal | Carbohydrates: 44g | Protein: 10g | Fat: 13g | Sodium: 139mg | Fiber: 2g | Calcium: 4mg

---

Low Fodmap Hard Shell Tacos

Serving size: 4   Prep Time: 15 mins
Cook Time: 15 mins   Total Time: 30 mins

INGREDIENTS

Tacos & Filling:

- 8 hard taco shells

- 1 tablespoon Garlic-Infused Oil, produced using vegetable oil, or bought equivalent.
- 1- pound (455 g) ground turkey, chicken or lean ground beef
- 2 teaspoons Gourmand Low FODMAP Taco Seasoning
- 1 teaspoon Gourmand Garlic Scape Powder
- ½ cup (32 g) chopped onions, green portions only ½ cup (75 g) chopped red bell pepper
- 3 tablespoons tomato paste
- 1/2 cup (120 ml) Organic Chicken Bone Broth or Organic Beef Bone Broth
- Kosher salt
- Freshly ground black pepper

Toppings:

- 1 cup (94 g) shredded green cabbage
- 1 cup (45 g) shredded Iceberg lettuce
- 1 medium carrot, peeled and grated ¼ cup (60 g) lactose-free sour cream or lactose-free plain yogurt
- ¼ cup (8 g) chopped cilantro
- 2 teaspoons freshly squeezed lime juice
- Pinch of sugar
- Kosher salt
- Freshly ground black pepper
- 120 g sliced avocado

- ¼ cup (30 g) crumbled cotija, or other low FODMAP cheese, such as cheddar or Monterey Jack
- Low FODMAP salsa

INSTRUCTIONS

1. Position oven rack to the center of the oven. Preheat the oven to 300°F. Wrap hard tortilla shells in aluminum foil and set in the oven while you prepare the filling.
2. For the Taco Filling: Heat vegetable oil based Garlic-Infused Oil in a large pan over medium heat. Add ground turkey, chicken or beef and cook until just beginning to brown, then add Gourmand Low FODMAP Taco Seasoning and Gourmand Garlic Scape Powder and keep breaking up the protein and tossing around until everything is blended and the protein is about halfway cooked through; this will just be a few minutes.
3. Add the chopped scallions and bell pepper and continue to sauté for a minute, then toss in tomato paste and stock and continue to simmer until protein is cooked through. Adjust salt and pepper to taste; keep heated.

4. For the Toppings: Toss together the cabbage, lettuce and carrots. Stir in sour cream or yogurt, cilantro, lime juice, and sugar. Season to taste with salt and pepper.

Assembly:

- Fill warmed taco shells with taco filling and top with cabbage slaw, diced avocado and crumbled cheese. Offer low FODMAP salsa on the side and dig down!

NUTRITION

Calories: 478 kcal | Carbohydrates: 27g | Protein: 37g | Fat: 26g | Saturated Fat: 2g | Polyunsaturated Fat: 2g | Monounsaturated Fat: 2g | Trans Fat: 0.1g | Cholesterol: 62 mg | Sodium: 230mg | Potassium: 512mg | Fiber: 5g | Sugar: 5g | Vitamin A: 215 IU | Vitamin C: 3mg | Calcium: 32mg | Iron: 2mg

---

Low FODMAP Eggplant Zucchini Tomato Pasta Sauce

Serving size: 6   Prep Time: 5 mins
Cook Time: 20 mins   Total Time: 25 mins

INGREDIENTS

- ¼ cup (60 ml) Garlic-Infused Oil, prepare with olive oil or bought equivalent, divided 1 pound (455 g) eggplant, trimmed and cut into ½-inch (12 mm) dice, with skin included
- Kosher salt
- Freshly ground black pepper
- 8- ounces (225 g) zucchini, trimmed and sliced into ½-inch (12 mm) dice
- ¼ cup (20 g) cut onions, green portions only 1, 14.5 ounce can (411 g) chopped tomatoes
- 3/4 teaspoon dried basil
- Parmesan, optional

INSTRUCTIONS

1. Heat a nonreactive big pan over medium heat; add roughly 1 ½ teaspoons of oil and cook until shimmering. Add about half of the eggplant, season with salt and pepper, and sauté until softened, browned and cooked through. Remove to a dish. Repeat with approximately 1 ½ teaspoons of the oil and the remainder of the eggplant, adding to the bowl when done.

2. Add remaining teaspoons of oil to the pan and sauté the zucchini and onions until the

zucchini is crisp tender. Add the eggplant back to the pan along with the tomatoes and basil. Cover and boil for approximately 5 minutes, stirring periodically. Taste and season with salt and pepper. Continue to boil for a few more minutes to develop flavor.

3. Meanwhile, cook your pasta and reserve a tiny amount of cooking water when you drain it. Toss the pasta with your sauce and a little conserved water to help the sauce cover the spaghetti. Serve immediately.

NUTRITION

Calories: 125 kcal | Carbohydrates: 10g | Protein: 2g | Fat: 10g | Saturated Fat: 1g | Sodium: 7mg | Potassium: 138mg | Fiber: 1g | Sugar: 2g | Vitamin A: 85 IU | Vitamin C: 6.8mg | Calcium: 25mg | Iron: 0.8mg

Bowl Of Orange Chicken And Broccoli With Low-fodmap

Serving size: 4   Prep Time: 20 mins
Cook Time 15 mins Total Time 35 mins

INGREDIENTS

- Sesame oil, one tablespoon equal
- 1 1/2 pounds of chicken thighs, chopped into pieces that are suitable for snacking
- One-half cup of Nourishing Vegetable Broth, which may be found on page 178 of the book, or low-FODMAP chicken broth
- 1 orange, with its zest and juice grated finely
- half a cup of brown sugar
- 1/4 cup soy sauce
- 3 cups broccoli florets, chopped into bite-size portions
- 3 cups sliced peeled carrots
- 1/4 cup sliced scallions, green parts only
- 2 teaspoons sesame seeds

INSTRUCTIONS

1. In a large skillet, heat the oil over medium heat. Add the chicken, and heat for 5 to 7 minutes, or until cooked through and browned. Remove from the heat.

2. In a small saucepan, mix together the broth, orange zest and juice, sugar, and soy sauce. Bring to a boil, then decrease the heat to a simmer, and cook for 8 to 10 minutes, or until thickened somewhat.

3. Pour the mixture over the chicken in the skillet. Mix thoroughly to coat.
4. In a medium saucepan, add the broccoli, carrots, and approximately ½ cup water. Place over medium-high heat, and cook for 5 minutes, or until tender. Divide into 4 bowls, then top with the chicken, scallions, and sesame seeds.

NUTRITION

Calories: 531 kcal | Carbohydrates: 24g | Protein: 32g | Fat: 34g | Saturated Fat: 8g | Cholesterol: 167 mg | Sodium: 968mg | Potassium: 632mg | Fiber: 4g | Sugar: 17g | Vitamin A: 558IU | Vitamin C: 61mg | Calcium: 99mg | Iron: 3mg

---

Low Fodmap Turkey Chili With Sweet Potato & Lentils

Serving size: 6 Total Time: 50 mins

INGREDIENTS
- 2 teaspoons garlic-infused olive oil
- ½ cup chopped leek leaves (dark green portions only)

- 1 pound lean ground turkey (I use 93% lean)
- 2 tablespoons tomato paste
- 2 cups low FODMAP chicken broth (or low FODMAP vegetarian broth)
- 2 cups (up to 300 grams) peeled and chopped sweet potato (approximately 2 medium sweet potatoes)
- 2 medium tomatoes, core removed and sliced (approximately 2 cups)
- 2 tablespoons low FODMAP taco seasoning
- 1 teaspoon ground cinnamon
- 1 (15-ounce) can lentils, drained and rinsed
- Salt and pepper

INSTRUCTIONS

1. Heat a Dutch oven or soup pot (with lid) over medium to medium-high heat. Once heated, add olive oil and leek leaves. Saute leek leaves till brilliant green, aromatic, and tender.

2. Add ground turkey and heat, breaking into crumbles, until nearly thoroughly browned. Once the turkey is nearly done, toss in the tomato paste and simmer approximately 1 minute longer.

3. Add the low FODMAP chicken broth, sweet potatoes, diced tomatoes, low FODMAP taco seasoning, and ground cinnamon to the turkey mixture and toss to blend. Adjust heat to high, and bring soup to a boil. Cover, lower heat to medium-low, and simmer for 12-15 minutes or until sweet potatoes are cooked.

4. Stir in drained and rinsed lentils and continue cooking until soup is cooked thoroughly. Season with salt and pepper.

5. Serve warm with optional toppings.

NUTRITION

Calories Per Serving: 304

Total Fat 11.4g Total Carbohydrate 28.6g 29%Dietary Fiber 8.2g 49%Protein 24.3g

---

Low Fodmap Pasta With Tuna & Sun Dried Tomatoes

Servings size: 6 Prep Time: 10 mins
Cook Time: 10 mins Total Time: 20 mins

INGREDIENTS

- 12 ounces (340 g) low FODMAP gluten-free pasta, such as farfalle, rigatoni, fusilli
- 2 tablespoons Garlic-Infused Oil, prepared with olive oil
- 1/3 cup (24 g) finely sliced scallions, green portions only
- 3/4 ounce (20 g) oil-packed sun dried tomatoes, drained and coarsely chopped (to equal approximately ⅓ cup)
- 2 medium tomatoes, cored and halved crosswise
- 2, (142 g) cans oil or water packed tuna, light or white, drained properly
- 1 tablespoon red wine vinegar
- Pinch of red pepper flakes
- 1/3 cup (12 g) finely cut fresh flat-leaf parsley
- 1 1/2 ounces (40 g) Parmesan cheese, shredded
- Kosher salt
- Freshly ground black pepper

INSTRUCTIONS

1. Bring a big saucepan of salted water to a boil. Meanwhile, heat a large pan over medium

heat and add the scallion greens and sun dried tomatoes and sauté for a minute then add the fresh tomatoes, tuna, vinegar and the red pepper flakes. Sauté around for a couple of minutes and keep warm while you complete the meal.

2. Cook the pasta until al dente. Remove ¼ cup (60 ml) of the starchy pasta water and save. Do not overcook the pasta since it will be placed in the skillet to cook as well.

3. Drain pasta thoroughly, then put the pasta to the pan, now over low-medium heat, and mix well with the sauce. By eye, add approximately half of the parsley and the Parmesan and keep tossing until the cheese is melted - this will happen in less than a minute. Add saved pasta water if, and only if, the sauce needs some liquid. Some tomatoes will be quite juicy and you may not need the water. Taste the sauce and season with salt and pepper as required. Divide the spaghetti in heated dishes and top with remaining parsley and Parmesan.

NUTRITION

Calories: 355 kcal | Carbohydrates: 45g | Protein: 24g | Fat: 10g | Saturated Fat: 1g | Sodium: 64mg | Potassium: 153mg | Fiber: 3g | Sugar: 1g | Vitamin A: 385 IU | Vitamin C: 9.2mg | Calcium: 4mg | Iron: 0.2mg

---

Low Fodmap Manicotti With Kale

Serving Size 6 Prep Time: 20 mins
Cook Time: 55 mins. Total Time: 1 hr 15 mins

INGREDIENTS

Pasta & Filling:

- 7- ounce (198 g) box low FODMAP gluten-free manicotti shells, such as Jovial
- 2 tablespoons Garlic-Infused Oil, prepared using olive oil, or bought product
- ¼ cup (16 g) chopped scallions, green portions only
- 3- ounces (85 g) baby kale, chopped 2 big eggs
- 15- ounces (425 g) low FODMAP ricotta
- 2/3 cup (65 g) grated Parmesan cheese

- 2- ounces (55 g) mozzarella, shredded ¼ cup (8 g) coarsely chopped flat-leaf parsley
- Kosher salt
- Freshly ground black pepper
- Pastry bag; I use disposable

Assembly & Topping:

- 3 cups (720 ml) low FODMAP marinara or tomato sauce, such as our Quick Tomato Sauce
- 8- ounces (225 g) mozzarella, shredded ¼ cup (25 g) grated Parmesan cheese

INSTRUCTIONS

1. Position rack in center of oven. Preheat the oven to 350°F (180°C). Have ready a 13-inch by 9-inch (33 cm by 23 cm) rectangular ceramic baking dish.
2. For the Pasta & Filling: Bring a big saucepan of salted water to a boil and cook the manicotti shells for 4 minutes, no longer. Drain.
3. Heat a large sauté pan over low-medium heat and sauté scallion greens for a few minutes until softened but not browned. Add the young greens and sauté for a minute or two until wilted. Set aside and cool.

4. Meanwhile, beat the eggs in a large mixing bowl then toss in the ricotta, Parmesan, mozzarella, parsley and cooled scallion/kale combination. Season liberally with salt and pepper.

Assembly & Topping:

1. Spread a substantial quantity of tomato sauce on the bottom of the dish to cover.

2. Scoop ricotta filling into a pastry bag and snip the bottom to form a 1/2-inch (12 mm) circular hole. Pick up the manicotti one at a time and pipe the filling into the manicotti, taking care not to over fill. Start placing the manicotti in the dish as you go using photos to aid you. Repeat with manicotti and filling and make a single layer of manicotti. For serving reasons it helps to recall your manicotti configuration.

3. Pour the remaining tomato sauce on top equally over the manicotti, then sprinkle with mozzarella and Parmesan. Cover with foil and bake for 40 minutes. Uncover, and continue baking for approximately 10 minutes longer or until the cheese has gently browned. Let settle for a couple of minutes and serve with a green salad.

NUTRITION

Calories: 780 kcal | Carbohydrates: 61g | Protein: 43g | Fat: 42g | Saturated Fat: 12g | Cholesterol: 69mg | Sodium: 869mg | Potassium: 81mg | Fiber: 1g | Sugar: 1g | Vitamin A: 632IU | Calcium: 639 mg | Iron: 1mg

SOUP RECIPES

Low Fodmap Carrot-ginger Soup

Servings size 8 Prep Time: 10 mins
Cook Time: 30 mins Total Time: 40 mins

INGREDIENTS

- 1 teaspoon extra-virgin olive oil or butter
- ½ cup roughly chopped fennel bulb
- 1 medium celery stalk, finely chopped
- 2 tablespoons grated peeled fresh ginger, plus more as required
- 6 cups Nourishing Vegetable Broth, from the book or use our Low FODMAP Vegetable Broth
- 6 medium carrots, peeled and finely chopped
- 2 medium yellow potatoes, finely chopped
- 1/4 teaspoon freshly ground black pepper + more as required
- ¼ teaspoon salt + more as required (optional)
- 1/2 cup vegan yogurt, optional

INSTRUCTIONS

1. In a big saucepan, heat the oil over medium-high heat. Add the fennel and celery,

and sauté for 5 minutes, or until softened. Reduce the heat to medium. Add the ginger, and simmer, stirring frequently, for 2 minutes.

2. Add the broth, carrots, potatoes, pepper, and salt (if using). Bring to a boil. Cover, lower the heat to a simmer, and cook for 15 to 20 minutes, or until the potatoes and carrots are fork-tender.

3. Using an immersion blender or a food processor, purée the soup. Taste, then season with extra grated ginger, salt, or pepper, if desired. Serve with additional pepper and a dollop of yogurt (if using) on top.

NUTRITION

Calories: 69 kcal | Carbohydrates: 14g | Protein: 1g | Fat: 1g | Sodium: 73mg | Fiber: 2g | Sugar: 3g

---

Low Fodmap Soba Miso Soup

Servings size 4 Prep Time: 10 mins
Cook Time: 20 mins Total Time: 30 mins

INGREDIENTS

- 4 large eggs, chilled; optional

- 4- ounces (115 g) soba noodles
- Kosher salt
- 2 tablespoons Low FODMAP Garlic-Infused Oil, prepared using vegetable oil, or bought equivalent
- 1 tablespoon toasted sesame oil
- 6- ounces (170 g) trimmed oyster mushrooms, torn off into separate portions
- 1 tablespoon low sodium gluten-free soy sauce
- 3 cups (720 ml) Low FODMAP Vegetable Broth 3 cups (720 ml) water
- 8- ounces (225 g) young bok choy, bottom root end chopped away
- ¼ cup (24 g) miso ¼ cup (16 g) sliced scallions, green parts only
- Sesame Seeds
- Sriracha

INSTRUCTIONS

1. Make the jammy eggs, if using. Have a basin of cold water placed aside. Bring a big saucepan of water to a boil, ensuring sure the level of the water will enable the eggs to immerse. Use a slotted spoon to drop the eggs into the water and adjust the heat to a low,

gradual boil and cook for precisely 6 ½ minutes. Remove eggs with a slotted spoon and dip into a dish of icy water. Allow to soak for approximately 1 minute, then remove and put aside on the counter.

2. Using the same pot, bring a large quantity of salted water to a boil over high heat and cook the soba noodles until al dente. Drain and rinse with cold water. Divide the noodles into 4 hot soup bowls. No need to clean the pot; you will use it again

3. While the soba is cooking, heat the Low FODMAP Garlic-Infused Oil and toasted sesame oil in a pan over medium heat. Add the mushrooms and sauté until softened. Add the soy sauce, then crank heat up a touch and make the mushrooms a bit crispy. Remove from heat and put aside.

4. Combine the Low FODMAP Vegetable Broth and water in the prepared pot and bring to a boil over high heat. Add the bok choy, adjust heat, and simmer for a few minutes or until the bok choy is crisp/tender. Remove from heat and rapidly whisk in the miso.

5. Divide miso soup and bok choy between bowls with noodles, top with mushrooms.

Peel eggs, slice in half, add to bowls, garnish with scallions and sesame seeds and serve immediately. Pass the Sriracha and limit it to 1 teaspoon (5 g) each serve.

NUTRITION

Calories: 331 kcal | Carbohydrates: 32g | Protein: 15g | Fat: 17g | Saturated Fat: 2g | Cholesterol: 211 mg | Sodium: 909 mg | Potassium: 181mg | Fiber: 2g | Sugar: 2g | Vitamin A: 2842IU | Vitamin C: 26mg | Calcium: 118mg | Iron: 3mg

---

Low FODMAP Chicken Enchilada Soup

Prep Time: 10 mins Total Time: 8 hrs 15 mins

INGREDIENTS

- 2 teaspoons garlic-infused olive oil
- ½ cup (45 grams) chopped leek leaves (green portions alone)
- 300 grams drained, canned tomatillos (about ½ of a 28 oz. can)
- ½ to 1 jalapeño, halved and seeds removed (optional)
- 1 teaspoon ground cumin

- 4 cups low FODMAP chicken broth
- 1 pound boneless, skinless chicken breasts
- 1 to 2 teaspoons lime juice
- ½ cup finely chopped fresh cilantro (optional)
- Salt and pepper

INSTRUCTIONS

1. Heat olive oil in a pan over medium heat. Saute leek leaves till brilliant green, aromatic, and tender. Place the sautéed leek leaves into a blender. Add tomatillos, jalapeño, cumin, and ¼ cup water. Blend until smooth.
2. Pour tomatillo mixture into a slow cooker. Add chicken broth. Stir to combine. Add chicken. Cover and cook for 6-8 hours on low or 3-4 hours on high.
3. Using a slotted spoon, take chicken from a slow cooker and shred. (I prefer to use two forks.) Return the shredded chicken back into the slow cooker and stir to combine. Add lime juice and optional cilantro. Adjust taste as required with salt and pepper.
4. Serve heated topped with optional toppings.

NUTRITION

Calories Per Serving: 248 % Total Fat 11.4g, Total Carbohydrate 8.5g, Dietary Fiber 1.9g 56% Protein 28.2g

---

Low Fodmap Vegetarian Sour Soup

INGREDIENTS

Soup:

- 2/3- ounce (19 g) dried wood ear fungus
- ¾- ounce (20 g) dried shiitake mushrooms
- Boiling Water
- 8 cups (2 L) low FODMAP vegetable broth, handmade, or Gourmand Organic Vegetable Broth
- 1 1/2 teaspoons gluten-free low sodium soy sauce, such as San-J
- 1 teaspoon toasted sesame oil
- 1 teaspoon ground white pepper preferably freshly ground
- 1/4 teaspoon sugar or to taste
- 1 fresh small red chile pepper, deseeded and diced, optional; or ½ teaspoon dried red chile flakes, or to taste
- 8- ounces (225 g) firm tofu, drained, sliced into cubes or little bite-sized portions

- 5- ounces (140 g) prepared bamboo shoots; canned or packed, cut strips, drained
- ¼ cup (60 ml) cup white vinegar, or to taste
- Kosher salt to taste

Thickener & Garnish

- ¼ cup (60 ml) water
- ¼ (32 g) cup cornstarch
- 1 big egg thoroughly beaten
- ¼ cup (16 g) chopped scallion greens

INSTRUCTIONS

1. For the Soup: Place the wood ears in one heatproof dish, and the shiitake in another. Cover each with boiling water. (I set a saucer on top of the shiitake to keep them submerged; the saucer is somewhat smaller than the bowl). Allow to sit for 1 hour. Drain both. (You may store the shiitake soaking water if you would want to utilize it for another usage; no assurance about FODMAP content). Chop the wood ear fungus into bit-sized pieces. Trim and remove any tough shiitake stems and discard. Thinly slice the shiitake mushroom tops.

2. Place the veggie broth in a large stock pot. Stir in the soy sauce, sesame oil, white

pepper, ¼ teaspoon sugar, and chopped chile or ½ teaspoon chile flakes. Bring to a simmer, then toss in the tofu, bamboo shoots, rehydrated wood ears and shiitake. Simmer for a few minutes, then whisk in vinegar. Taste and add salt, if required.

3. This is your chance to balance the tastes. Need more heat? More sweet? More sour? Simple season to your liking.

Thickener & Garnish:

- Combine the water and cornstarch to produce a slurry. Stir your boiling soup so that it is swirling, then sprinkle in the cornstarch slurry. Simmer for another 30 seconds to thicken. Stir again to produce that swirl and drizzle in the beaten egg. It will cook practically immediately. Soup is ready to serve with scallion green garnish.

NUTRITION

Calories: 99 kcal | Carbohydrates: 12g | Protein: 6g | Fat: 4g | Saturated Fat: 0.2g | Polyunsaturated Fat: 0.1g | Monounsaturated Fat: 0.2g | Trans Fat: 0.003g | Cholesterol: 23 mg | Sodium: 10mg | Potassium: 50mg | Fiber: 0.4g | Sugar: 0.3g | Vitamin A: 34IU | Vitamin C: 0.1mg | Calcium: 5mg | Iron: 0.2mg

Low Fodmap Spicy Smoky Pumpkin Soup

Serving size: 6 Prep Time:10 mins
Cook Time:15 mins Total Time:25 mins

INGREDIENTS

Soup:

- 2 tablespoons unsalted butter, sliced into pieces
- 1 tablespoon Garlic-Infused Oil, produced with olive oil, or bought equivalent
- 3/4 cup chopped onions, green bits only
- 1/2 teaspoon smoked paprika
- 1/4 teaspoon cinnamon
- 1/4 teaspoon nutmeg
- 1/8 teaspoon cayenne or to taste
- 3 cups (720 ml) water
- 2 tablespoons Fody Chicken Soup Base or Vegetable Soup Base
- 1, 15- ounce (425 g) can pure pumpkin, such as Libby's
- 1 tablespoon firmly packed light brown sugar
- 1 teaspoon kosher salt

- 3/4 cup (180 ml) lactose-free half and half, optional, and more as required
- Freshly ground black pepper

INSTRUCTIONS

1. Heat a medium sized saucepan over low-medium heat, add butter and oil and simmer until melted. Add scallions and sauté a few minutes, stirring periodically until tender. Add smoked paprika, cinnamon, nutmeg, and ⅛ teaspoon cayenne and sauté 15 seconds longer.

2. Add water and soup base and mix together thoroughly. Alternatively you may use 3 cups (720 ml) of either or Low FODMAP Chicken Stock or Vegetable Broth. Then stir in canned pumpkin, brown sugar and salt. Bring to a boil and cook for approximately 10 minutes, whisking periodically. Cool slightly, add half & half, if needed and then purée in a blender until silky smooth. Taste, add pepper and adjust salt, if required. Soup is ready to serve; reheat if required.

3. You may thin it down a bit more, if you prefer, using water, additional half-and half or chicken or vegetable stock. If you want to

make it a little fancier, whisk up a little lactose-free sour cream and pour on top and/or sprinkle on a few toasted pepitas. Soup may also be chilled and then refrigerated in an airtight container for up to 4 days.

NUTRITION

Calories: 143 kcal | Carbohydrates: 9g | Protein: 3g | Fat: 11g | Saturated Fat: 1g | Sodium: 394mg | Fiber: 2g | Sugar: 4g | Vitamin A: 80IU | Calcium: 4mg

---

Low Fodmap Shrimp & Corn Chowder

Servings size: 6 Prep Time: 10 mins
Cook Time: 30 mins

INGREDIENTS

- 2 fresh cobs of sweet corn
- 2 tablespoons Onion-Infused Oil, prepared using olive oil, or bought equivalent
- ½ cup (32 g) chopped scallions, green bits only 6 cups (1.4 L) Low FODMAP Vegetable Broth 12- ounces (340 g) Yukon Gold,

yellow-skinned or red-skinned waxy potatoes, diced

- 4 plum tomatoes, cored and cut
- 1 carrot, trimmed and cleaned, sliced in half crosswise ½ stalk celery, cut in half crosswise
- 1 tablespoon minced fresh basil, plus extra Kosher salt
- Freshly ground black pepper
- ½ pound (225 g) fresh shrimp peeled and deveined ½ medium zucchini, trimmed and sliced

INSTRUCTIONS

1. Shuck the corn and discard the husks and silk. Cut the corn from the cob, retaining any liquids and the kernels. Save the cobs.
2. Heat the oil in a large stockpot over low heat and add the onions. Sauté for a few minutes until softened. Add the corn cobs to the saucepan along with Vegetable Broth, potatoes, tomatoes, carrot, celery and 1 tablespoon chopped fresh basil. Bring to a boil, cover, and cook for 20 minutes or until. Potatoes should be soft and the flavors will have come together. Taste and season with some salt and pepper, if desired.

3. Remove and discard the corncobs, and carrot and celery bits. Add the shrimp and zucchini along with corn kernels and any liquids. Bring back to a simmer and cook just until zucchini is soft and shrimp has become opaque. Soup is ready to serve, topped with more fresh basil.

4. Soup may be chilled and stored for up to 3 days in an airtight container.

NUTRITION

Calories: 188 kcal | Carbohydrates: 25g | Protein: 11g | Fat: 7g | Saturated Fat: 1g | Cholesterol: 95mg | Sodium: 1246mg | Potassium: 264mg | Fiber: 2g | Sugar: 3g | Vitamin A: 504IU | Vitamin C: 8mg | Calcium: 72mg | Iron: 3mg

---

Salmon Chowder With Low Fodmap Dose

Serving size: 4 Prep: 5 mins
Cooking Time: 25 mins Total Time: 30 mins

INGREDIENTS

- 2 teaspoons of liquid Low in FODMAP Infused with Onion Oil or extra-virgin olive oil
- 1 cup (64 g) One-half cup (36 grammes) of cut scallions, only the green parts finely chopped leeks, green bits only 4 cups (960 ml) UHT unsweetened coconut milk
- 2 cups (480 ml) low FODMAP stock - fish (clam) or chicken
- 1- pound (455 g) celeriac, peeled and cut into big dice
- 1- pound (455 g) Yukon gold potatoes, peeled and cut into big dice
- 3 medium carrots, trimmed, peeled and sliced crosswise into ½-inch rounds
- 1 bay leaf ½ teaspoon dried thyme
- 1- pound (455 g) peeled salmon, ideally Atlantic, sliced into big pieces
- Kosher salt
- Freshly ground black pepper

INSTRUCTIONS

1. Heat oil in a large soup pot or Dutch oven over low-medium heat until it shimmers. Add scallion and leek greens and sauté until

softened but not browned, just a few minutes, then add coconut milk, stock, celeriac and potato cubes, carrots, bay leaf and thyme and whisk everything together thoroughly. Bring to a boil and cook until celeriac and potatoes are cooked, approximately 10 minutes.

2. Add the fish and continue to boil until the fish is opaque and cooked through; this will take around 5 minutes. Taste and season with salt and pepper; serve immediately.

NUTRITION

Calories: 569 kcal | Carbohydrates: 47g | Protein: 33g | Fat: 30g | Saturated Fat: 1g | Sodium: 1mg | Fiber: 3g | Sugar: 5g | Iron: 1mg

---

Low Fodmap Fish Chowder

Servings size: 6. Prep Time: 10 mins
Cook Time: 20 mins. Total Time: 30 mins

INGREDIENTS

- 2- ounces (55 g) slab bacon, rind removed, chopped
- 1 tablespoon unsalted butter

- 1/2 cup (36 g) coarsely sliced leeks, green parts only
- 2 medium carrots, trimmed, peeled and chopped
- 2 medium parsnips, trimmed, peeled and chopped
- 1 stalk celery, trimmed and diced
- 1 1/2 tablespoons fresh thyme leaves
- 2 cups (480 ml) bottled clam juice
- 1 cup (240 ml) water
- 1- pound (445 g) russet baking potatoes, peeled and sliced into big bite-sized portions
- 1 huge bay leaf 1 ¼ pounds (570 g) mild white fish filets, such as haddock, cod, hake or monkfish
- 1 cup (240 ml) lactose-free heavy cream, at room temperature
- Freshly ground black pepper
- Finely chopped fresh flat leaf parsley; optional
- Snipped fresh chives; optional

INSTRUCTIONS

1. Place bacon in a large, heavy Dutch oven and cook over low-medium heat to render the fat and cook until bacon is crisp. Remove bacon

pieces and reserve, draining on paper towels. Add butter and chopped leeks and sauté gently over low-medium heat for approximately 3 to 5 minutes or until leeks are tender but not browned. Add the carrots, parsnips, celery and thyme and sauté for approximately 1 minute to coat.

2. Add the clam juice, water, potatoes and bay leaf to the saucepan. Cover and boil for approximately 15 minutes or until the root veggies are completely tender. Use the back of a wooden spoon or a potato masher to mash some of the root vegetables directly in the kettle. Their starch will lend richness to the chowder.

3. Add the saved bacon, fish and the cream and simmer over low heat until the fish is cooked through and flaky, but do not allow the chowder to boil. Taste and add pepper as required. Soup is ready to serve but improves after it rests for an hour.

4. Serve with parsley and chives sprinkled on top, if preferred. The un-garnished chowder may be refrigerated overnight and warmed very gently without simmering or boiling.

NUTRITION

Calories: 434 kcal | Carbohydrates: 27g | Protein: 27g | Fat: 18g | Saturated Fat: 1g | Sodium: 7mg | Potassium: 194mg | Fiber: 4g | Sugar: 4g | Vitamin A: 24IU | Vitamin C: 10mg | Calcium: 21mg | Iron: 1mg

---

Low Fodmap Vegetable, Pasta & Bean Soup

Serving size: 14 Prep Time: 15 mins
Cook Time: 30 mins Total Time: 45 mins

INGREDIENTS
- 2 teaspoons of liquid Garlic-Infused Oil, produced using olive oil, or bought equal
- 3/4 cup (48 g) finely sliced scallions, green portions only 1/4 cup (18 g) finely sliced leeks, green portions only 8 cups (2 L) water
- 1, 28- ounce (794 g) can crushed tomatoes
- 1, 15.5- ounce (439 g) can chickpeas, drained, washed and drained again
- 12- ounces (340 g) chopped butternut squash
- 8- ounces (225 g) red potatoes, cleaned and chopped into little bite-sized chunks

- 6- ounces (170 g) cleaned and trimmed kale, cut finely
- 3 medium carrots, cleansed, trimmed and sliced into thick rounds (1/2-inch/12 mm or even bigger)
- 2 cups (150 g) chopped bok choy
- 1 medium patty pan or yellow squash cleaned, trimmed and sliced into thick rounds (approximately 1/2-inch/12 mm thick)
- 1 medium zucchini washed, trimmed, quartered and sliced into little bite-sized pieces
- 1 teaspoon dried basil
- 1 teaspoon smoked paprika
- 1 teaspoon dried thyme
- Kosher salt
- Freshly ground black pepper
- 1 cup (100 g) uncooked gluten-free elbow or tiny shell shaped pasta

INSTRUCTIONS

1. Place Garlic-Infused Oil in a big heavy saucepan or Dutch oven and heat over medium heat. Add onion and leek greens and sauté for a few minutes until tender. Add water, tinned tomatoes, chickpeas, squash,

potatoes, kale, carrots, bok choy, yellow squash, zucchini, basil, smoky paprika and thyme and toss everything together thoroughly. Season with salt and pepper.

2. Cover and bring to a boil over medium-high heat, then decrease heat down and simmer for at least 30 minutes or until veggies are cooked, stirring periodically. Taste and adjust seasoning as required.

3. Meanwhile, prepare pasta in a substantial quantity of salted water until al dente; drain and pour into soup (see Tips). Soup is ready to serve, or cool to room temperature and stored in an airtight container for up to 5 days. Freeze for up to 1 month, adding spaghetti when warming. Reheat as required.

NUTRITION

Calories: 142 kcal | Carbohydrates: 31g | Protein: 5g | Fat: 3g | Saturated Fat: 1g | Sodium: 7mg | Potassium: 3mg | Fiber: 3g | Sugar: 2g | Vitamin A: 70IU | Calcium: 7mg | Iron: 0.2mg

Low Fodmap Bouillabaisse

Serving size: 6 Prep Time: 15 mins
Cook Time: 45 mins Total Time: 1 hour

INGREDIENTS

Roasted Red Pepper Aioli:

- 1 big pasteurized egg yolk, at room temperature
- 2 tablespoons freshly squeezed lemon juice
- 1 teaspoon cold water
- ¼ teaspoon Dijon mustard
- Kosher salt
- 1 cup (240 ml) Garlic-Infused Oil, produced using olive oil, or bought equal
- ½ cup (85 g) very finely chopped, drained canned roasted red peppers
- Cayenne pepper
- Freshly ground black pepper
- Toast: 1, low FODMAP French baguette
- 2 teaspoons of liquid Garlic-Infused Oil, prepared using olive oil, or equivalent

Bouillabaisse:

- ¾ pound (340 g) big (26 to 30 count) shrimp, deveined, shells on ¼ cup (60 ml)

Garlic-Infused Oil, produced using olive oil, or bought equal

- 1 cup (140 g) finely sliced leeks, green portions only 1 cup (98 g) thinly sliced fresh fennel bulb; retain some fennel fronds (the delicate, feathery tips)
- 3 canned plum tomatoes, drained of liquid, diced
- 2 tablespoons chopped fresh flat-leaf parsley
- 2 tablespoons finely grated orange zest
- 1 teaspoon chopped fresh thyme
- ½ teaspoon fennel seeds, crushed 24 small to medium-size clams or mussels or ideally a mix of both, cleaned clear of sand and grit; debeard a mussels if required
- 1½ pounds (680 g) white flesh fish, ideally more than one species, such as cod filets, cod loins, red snapper, halibut, haddock, monkfish, or striped bass, cut into pieces
- ¾ pound (340 g) sea scallops; cut in half if extremely big
- 1 tablespoon chopped fresh basil
- Kosher salt
- Freshly ground black pepper

INSTRUCTIONS

For the Aioli:

1. Place the pasteurized egg yolk, lemon juice, cold water, mustard, and ½ teaspoon of salt in a medium-size nonreactive bowl. Whisk vigorously until mixed. Very gently, drop by drop, mix in approximately a quarter of the olive oil, stirring all the while. This will take many minutes; proceed gently, allowing the mayonnaise to thicken. Gradually add the remaining olive oil until the required thickness is obtained; you may not need all the oil, but you will most likely use at least ¾ cup (180 ml). Gently mix in the chopped peppers and cayenne to taste.

2. Season to taste with additional salt and with black pepper, if preferred. The aioli is ready to use, or chill in an airtight container for up to 2 days.

3. For the Toast: Right before starting to cook the shellfish, slice the bread into 1-inch (2.5 cm) slices, toast in a toaster or on a baking sheet in a 400°F (200°C) oven, then spray with the olive oil; put aside.

For the Bouillabaisse:

1. Peel the shrimp and lay them aside, retaining shells. Place the shells in a medium-size pot with 4½ cups (1 L) of water. Bring to a boil,

decrease the heat, and simmer for 5 minutes. This is a super-quick shellfish stock.

2. While the shrimp shells are simmering, heat the oil in a deep 5-quart (4.7 L) pot, such as a Dutch oven, over medium heat. Add the leek greens and sliced fennel and sauté for 3 to 5 minutes, or until softened but not browned.

3. Strain and measure out 4 cups (960 ml) of the stock for the bouillabaisse. Discard the shells. Add the shrimp stock, tomatoes, parsley, orange zest, thyme, and fennel seeds to the leek combination. Cover, raise the heat, and simmer for 10 minutes

4. Add the clams and/or mussels, cover, and simmer for approximately 5 minutes, or until the shells open, discarding any that do not open. Add the white fish and scallops, cover, and simmer for approximately 5 minutes, or until the fish is nearly opaque. Add the shrimp and simmer, covered, for approximately 3 to 5 minutes longer, or just until the shrimp become pink. Gently whisk in the basil and taste the broth. Season with salt and pepper, if preferred.

5. Place a piece or two of garlic bread in each bowl and top the toasts with a liberal dollop

of aioli. Ladle the stew on top and garnish with fennel fronds, if you prefer. Serve immediately

NUTRITION

Calories: 1116 kcal | Carbohydrates: 20g | Protein: 78g | Fat: 70g | Sodium: 123mg | Fiber: 1g | Sugar: 2g | Calcium: 30mg

---

Low Fodmap Cream, Tomato Soup With Grilled Cheese Croutons

Serving size: 3 Prep Time: 15 mins
Cook Time: 25 mins Total Time: 40 mins

INGREDIENTS

Soup:

- 2 teaspoons of liquid Low FODMAP Onion-Infused Oil, produced using olive oil, or bought equivalent
- 1 cup (64 g) cut scallions, green portions only
- 2, 28- ounce (794 g) cans of whole, peeled tomatoes in juice
- ½ teaspoon kosher salt, plus extra ¼ teaspoon freshly ground black pepper, plus extra 1/3

cup (75 ml) lactose-free half-and-half, or heavy cream

Grilled Cheese Croutons:

- 4 pieces of low FODMAP sliced bread ¼ cup (56 g) mayonnaise
- 2 tablespoons unsalted butter, softened 4-ounces (115 g) cheddar cheese, white or orange, Monterey Jack or a mix, at room temperature, cut very thinly

INSTRUCTIONS

For the Soup:

1. Heat oil over low-medium heat in a large Dutch-oven or heavy pot until it shimmers. Add scallion greens and sauté until softened but not browned. Add tomatoes and juice and smash tomatoes with your hands (fun but dirty) or squash with a potato masher. Either way proceed gently and look out for squirts! Add salt and pepper, bring to a boil, then decrease heat to a simmer, cover pot, and cook for 15 minutes. Taste and adjust seasoning.

2. Carefully transfer to blender and purée, or purée directly in the saucepan if you have an immersion blender. You may leave as is, or

for a more traditional texture, strain through a fine-meshed strainer (my choice) and return to the saucepan to reheat. Add cream, heat slowly, but do not boil. Keep warm.

For the Grilled Cheese Croutons:

1. You create the grilled cheese while the soup is cooking to save time, if you wish to multitask.

2. Lay the bread out on your work area in front of you and apply a spoonful of mayonnaise on each piece, edge to edge, coating fully.

3. Place a big nonstick or cast-iron pan on the stove over low heat and add butter. Melt the butter and swirl it around the pan. Place two pieces of bread in the pan, mayo side down. Divide cheese between the two pieces of bread and top with remaining bread, mayo side up. Increase heat to low-medium. Cook until the bottom is golden brown, turn and continue frying till the second side is similarly crispy and golden and the cheese has melted.

4. Pour heated soup into warm bowls. Cut sandwiches into little square "croutons", approximately 1-inch (2.5 cm) across. Divide croutons into dishes and serve immediately

NUTRITION

Calories: 524 kcal | Carbohydrates: 48g | Protein: 13g | Fat: 47g | Saturated Fat: 2g | Cholesterol: 8mg | Sodium: 744 mg | Sugar: 14g

---

Low Fodmap Summer Squash Soup

Servings size: 4 Prep Time: 10 mins
Cook Time: 30 mins Total Time: 40 mins

INGREDIENTS

- 3 tablespoons Garlic-Infused Oil, produced using vegetable oil or olive oil, or bought equivalent
- 1 cup (64 g) finely sliced scallions, green portions only
- 4 cups (600 g) chopped trimmed patty pan squash
- 4 medium Yukon gold potatoes, peeled and diced
- 3 medium carrots, trimmed, peeled and chopped
- 1 teaspoon cumin powder
- 1 teaspoon coriander

- 1 teaspoon turmeric
- 1 teaspoon paprika, plus additional for garnish
- 1/4 teaspoon mustard powder
- 1/4 teaspoon cinnamon
- 4 1/2 cups (1 L) Low FODMAP Vegetable Broth
- 3/4 cup (180 ml) canned full coconut milk, at room temperature
- Kosher salt
- Freshly ground black pepper
- Cilantro leaves

INSTRUCTIONS

1. Heat a big, heavy-bottomed pot over low-medium heat. Add the oil and the scallion greens and sauté until softened, but not browned. Add the squash, potatoes, carrots and all of the seasonings. Stir together and heat for a few minutes or until veggies just begin to soften. Add the stock, cover, bring to a boil, then lower heat and simmer for approximately 15 minutes or until all the veggies are very soft.

2. If you have an immersion blender, you can purée the soup directly in the saucepan.

Otherwise, move to a blender and purée. Return soup to pot, if required. Taste and season with salt and pepper. Soup is ready to garnish and serve. Divide the heated soup into serving dishes, swirl in some coconut milk, decorate with cilantro leaves and a sprinkling of paprika. You may also chill the puréed soup in an airtight container (before garnishing) for up to 4 days.

NUTRITION

Calories: 292 kcal | Carbohydrates: 43g | Protein: 6g | Fat: 10g | Saturated Fat: 1g | Cholesterol: 9mg | Sodium: 12mg | Potassium: 749 mg | Fiber: 5g | Sugar: 4g | Vitamin A: 246IU | Vitamin C: 33mg | Calcium: 25mg | Iron: 2mg

SALAD RECIPES

Low Fodmap Mediterranean Tuna Salad With Chickpeas

Servings size: 10 Prep Time: 5 minutes

INGREDIENTS

- 1, 15.5- ounce (439 g) can chickpeas drained, washed, drained and wiped dry
- 2, 5- ounce (142 g) cans light tuna, water-packed, drained thoroughly
- 1/2 cup (32 g) chopped scallions green parts only 2 medium (300 g) beefsteak tomato, cored and chopped 1 cup (150 g) sliced hothouse or seedless cucumber (keep skin on)
- Your Favorite Low FODMAP vinaigrette we propose an olive oil and vinegar based
- Oregano, dried or fresh chopped Kosher salt
- Freshly ground black pepper

INSTRUCTIONS

1. Gently whisk together the drained chickpeas, tuna, onions, tomatoes and cucumber. Dress gently with vinaigrette and season with oregano, salt and pepper to taste.

2. Ready to eat or may be refrigerated in an airtight container for up to 3 days.

NUTRITION

Calories: 114 kcal | Carbohydrates: 15g | Protein: 10g | Fat: 2g | Saturated Fat: 1g | Sodium: 14mg | Potassium: 136mg | Fiber: 4g | Sugar: 3g | Vitamin A: 15IU | Vitamin C: 0.6mg | Calcium: 23 mg | Iron: 1.4mg

---

Low Fodmap Pineapple Chicken Salad

Serving size: 8 Prep Time: 10 mins
Total Time: 10 mins

INGREDIENTS

- 2 cups (280 g) gently packed diced or shredded, cooked chicken
- 1 cup (140 g) chopped fresh pineapple
- ⅓ to 1/2 cup (75 g to 113 g) mayonnaise
- ½ cup (32 g) sliced scallions, green parts only
- 1 big stalk celery, 80 g total, chopped
- 1 teaspoon freshly squeezed lemon juice
- Kosher salt
- Freshly ground black pepper

- 2 teaspoons minced fresh tarragon, or ½ teaspoon dried; optional
- ¼ cup (25 g) gently toasted pecan halves, diced; optional

INSTRUCTIONS

1. In a large bowl, combine the chicken, pineapple, ⅓ cup (75 g) mayonnaise, onions, celery and lemon juice mixing the ingredients together until thoroughly combined. Use extra mayo if required. Taste and season with salt and pepper, then fold in the tarragon and/or pecans if using.
2. The salad is ready to serve or store in an airtight container for up to 3 days. We enjoy this equally on low FODMAP sandwich bread or on a bed of lettuce.

NUTRITION

Calories: 156 kcal | Carbohydrates: 5g | Protein: 10g | Fat: 11g | Saturated Fat: 1g | Cholesterol: 4mg | Sodium: 63mg | Fiber: 1g | Sugar: 1g | Vitamin A: 6IU

Low Fodmap Green Goddess Chicken Salad

Servings size: 4 Prep Time: 5 mins

INGREDIENTS

- 12 ounces (340 g) cooked chicken, dark or white flesh, no skin, either chopped into tiny cubes or shredded
- 1/4 cup (16 g) finely cut scallions, green bits only 1/2 cup (120 ml) Low FODMAP Green Goddess Dressing

INSTRUCTIONS

- Simply blend all the ingredients together until fully incorporated.
- Stuff into a sandwich or serve as a salad, maybe with some crunchy low FODMAP dippers and scoopers like pretzels, corn chips or carrot sticks.

NUTRITION

Calories: 191 kcal | Carbohydrates: 1g | Protein: 17g | Fat: 13g

Low Fodmap Chopped Chicken Caesar Salad

Servings size: 4 Prep Time: 10 mins
Cook Time: 5 mins Total Time: 15 mins

INGREDIENTS

- 1 1/2 teaspoons unsalted butter
- 1 1/2 teaspoons Garlic-Infused Oil, prepared with olive oil or bought equivalent, such as FODY Garlic-Infused Olive Oil
- 2, 1/2- inch (12 ml) thick slices of low FODMAP sourdough bread from an 8-inch (20 cm round loaf), cubed or 3 slices low FODMAP gluten-free sliced sandwich bread, such as Udi's, cubed 2 big heads of Romaine lettuce hard root end removed, leaves cut into bite-sized pieces to produce 8 cups
- 1 entire chicken breast (1 pound total/455 g), cooked - poached, roasted, grilled - your option!, sliced into bite-sized pieces
- 3/4 cup (180 ml) Low FODMAP Caesar Salad Dressing
- Kosher salt
- Freshly ground black pepper
- 1- ounce (30 g) big shavings of Parmesan cheese, optional

INSTRUCTIONS

- Place butter and Garlic-Infused Oil in a large nonstick pan and melt over medium heat. Add cubed bread and stir them around to coat in the grease. Cook over medium heat, turning the cubes regularly until gently toasted and golden brown, approximately 3 minutes total. Set aside.

- Toss the chopped lettuce and chicken together in a large mixing dish and add just enough Low FODMAP Caesar Salad Dressing to moisten gently. Taste and adjust seasoning, if required. Toss in croutons and additional shavings of Parmesan flakes, if using. Salad is ready to serve and should be served immediately or it will go soggy.

NUTRITION

Calories: 467 kcal | Carbohydrates: 16g | Protein: 47g | Fat: 23g | Sodium: 424mg | Fiber: 3g | Sugar: 3g | Calcium: 15mg

Low Fodmap Asian Salad

Serving size: 8 Prep Time: 15 mins

INGREDIENTS

Peanut Butter Dressing:

- 6 tablespoons (102 g) peanut butter, either natural or no-stir style
- 3 tablespoons firmly packed light brown sugar
- 3 tablespoons rice vinegar or apple cider vinegar
- 3 tablespoons low-sodium gluten-free soy sauce
- 11/2 teaspoons fish sauce, such as Red Boat brand
- 1 1/2 teaspoons freshly squeezed lime juice
- 1 1/2 tablespoons Garlic-Infused Oil, produced with vegetable oil or bought equivalent ¼ to ½ teaspoon sambal oelek other low FODMAP spicy sauce such as Tabasco, or more to taste
- Water, if required

Chicken Salad:

- 1- pound (455 g) shredded cooked chicken heated or at room temperature

- 4 cups (356 g) finely shredded green cabbage
- 2 medium carrots, trimmed and grated
- 1 red bell pepper, cored and finely sliced
- 2 Persian cucumbers, ends removed, cut into big julienne
- 1/2 cup (16 g) chopped fresh cilantro, divided
- 1/2 cup (80 g) chopped roasted peanuts, split
- 1/2 cup (32 g) sliced scallions, green portions only, split

INSTRUCTIONS

1. For the Peanut Butter Dressing: Combine peanut butter, brown sugar, vinegar, soy sauce, fish sauce, lime juice, oil and spicy sauce in a blender and mix until smooth and blended. Scrape down the blender as required. Taste and apply extra spicy sauce if desired. If you use natural peanut butter and the mixture is a touch thick, blend in a tablespoon or two of water. You want a flowable texture. The dressing may be prepared a day ahead and refrigerated in an airtight container.

2. For Chicken Salad Assembly: In a large mixing bowl, combine together the chicken, cabbage, carrot, bell pepper, cucumbers of the

cilantro, half the peanuts and half of the scallions (you may do this by eye). Add part of the dressing and toss to coat. Only pour enough dressing to gently cover the salad components. You may not need all of the sauce. Serve garnished with leftover cilantro, peanuts and scallions. Salad may be presented with the chicken slightly warm, or everything at room temperature.

3. Salad may be refrigerated in an airtight container for up to 3 days. Bring to room temperature before serving. It is great if you can garnish with the scallions, peanuts and cilantro immediately before serving. Or even better, if you know you want to prepare well ahead, keep salad and dressing separate until close to serving time (and those garnishes, too!)

NUTRITION

Calories: 314 kcal | Carbohydrates: 15g | Protein: 24g | Fat: 19g | Saturated Fat: 1g | Cholesterol: 43mg | Sodium: 1026mg | Potassium: 130mg | Fiber: 3g | Sugar: 8g | Vitamin A: 25 IU | Calcium: 7mg | Iron: 0.7mg

Warm Bacon & Avocado Salad

Serving size: 8   Prep Time: 10 mins
Cook Time: 10 mins   Total Time: 20 mins

INGREDIENTS

Salad:

- Selection of lettuces and salad greens, such as butterhead, iceberg, Belgian endive, radicchio, , watercress, and salad burnet
- 6- ounces (170 g) slab bacon, unsmoked or mildly smoked
- Clarified butter, or a blend of butter and oil, plus olive oil, for frying the bacon
- 4 slices low FODMAP white bread
- Sunflower or olive oil, for frying the croutons
- 1 avocado (160 g total)
- 18 fresh walnut halves, to garnish (optional)
- Dressing:
- 3 tablespoons walnut oil, or a blend of 2 teaspoons walnut oil and 1 tablespoon sunflower oil
- 1 tablespoon Chardonnay wine vinegar
- 1 teaspoon freshly chopped chives
- 1 teaspoon freshly cut flat-leaf parsley

- Sea salt and freshly ground black pepper

INSTRUCTIONS

1. Wash and dry the salad greens, then shred into bite-size pieces. Put into a bowl, cover, and chill until required.

2. Cut the skin from the bacon, then cut the bacon into ¼-inch (6 mm) cubes. In a skillet, fry in clarified butter or a combination of butter and oil until browned. Drain on paper towels.

3. Make the Croutons: Cut the crusts off the bread, then cut into strips ¼ inch (6 mm) broad and into precise cubes. In a skillet, heat at least ¾ inch (2 cm) sunflower or olive oil until nearly smoking. Add the croutons to the heated oil and toss once or twice; they will brown nearly instantly. Place a strainer over a Pyrex or stainless steel bowl. When the croutons are golden brown, pour the oil and croutons into the sieve. Drain the croutons on paper towels. The croutons may be prepared many hours or even a day ahead.

Make the Dressing:

1. In a small bowl, whisk together the liquid ingredients, then add the chopped herbs and season with salt and freshly ground pepper.
2. Halve the avocado and remove the pit. Peel and cut into ½-inch (12 mm) dice.
3. To serve, mix the salad leaves with just enough of the dressing to make them sparkle. Add the crisp, toasty croutons and the cubed avocado. Toss lightly and divide the salad among eight dishes. In a heated pan, recook the bacon in a splash of olive oil until crisp and golden, then spread the hot bacon over the salad. Garnish with the walnut halves, if desired. Serve straight away.

NUTRITION
Calories: 246 kcal | Carbohydrates: 9g | Protein: 5g | Fat: 21g | Saturated Fat: 1g | Fiber: 2g | Sugar: 1g

---

Low Fodmap Brussels Sprouts Salad

8 Servings size: 8 Prep Time: 10 mins
Total Time: 10 minutes

INGREDIENTS

Salad:

- 10- ounces (280 g) fresh Brussels sprouts, cut to match 8-ounces (225 g) and shredded
- 1 big head Romaine lettuce, cored and shredded, (approximately 5 to 6-ounces)
- ½ cup (69 g) toasted whole smoked almonds, chopped ½ cup (87 g) pomegranate seeds
- ¼ cup (8 g) chopped fresh flat leaf parsley

Dressing:

- 1/3 cup (75 ml) extra virgin olive oil
- 1/3 cup (75 ml) freshly squeezed lemon juice
- 2 tablespoons Dijon mustard
- 2 tablespoons maple syrup; optional
- Kosher salt
- Freshly ground black pepper
- Shaved Parmesan; optional

INSTRUCTIONS

Salad

1. Toss together all of the salad ingredients in a serving dish.

For the Dressing & Assembly

1. Shake the oil, lemon juice, maple syrup (if using) and mustard together in a closed container. Season to taste with salt and

pepper. Dress the salad, gently, yet thoroughly (you could have dressing leftover). Salad is ready to serve but really improves if let to stand for 1 hour. Garnish with shaved Parmesan, if preferred.

NUTRITION

Calories: 148 kcal | Carbohydrates: 8g | Protein: 3g | Fat: 13g | Saturated Fat: 1g | Sodium: 15mg | Potassium: 35mg | Fiber: 1g | Sugar: 3g | Vitamin C: 2mg | Calcium: 3mg | Iron: 1mg

---

Low Fodmap Tuna Salad

Servings size: 6 Prep Time: 5 mins

INGREDIENTS

- 2, 5-ounce (142 g) cans tuna, ideally water packed 3/4 cup (60 g), chopped bok choy stems, OR 3/4 cup (113 g), diced European hothouse cucumber, OR 1/2 medium (10 g) celery stalk, diced 2/3 cup (150 g) mayonnaise
- 1 1/2 teaspoons lemon juice
- 1/2 teaspoon dried dill

- Freshly ground black pepper

INSTRUCTIONS

1. Scrape the tuna into a wire-mesh strainer placed over a bowl and press out as much liquid as possible, using the back of a wooden spoon; don't hold back! Discard the liquid. Place the tuna in a mixing bowl, toss in the chopped vegetable of choice (just one of them!), mayonnaise, lemon juice, dill (to taste) and then liberally season to taste with pepper.

2. The tuna is ready to use in sandwiches or as part of a salad dish. May be refrigerated for up to 3 days in an airtight container.

NUTRITION

Calories: 279 kcal | Carbohydrates: 2g | Protein: 18g | Fat: 22g | Saturated Fat: 3g | Cholesterol: 11mg | Sodium: 204mg | Fiber: 1g | Sugar: 1g | Vitamin A: 15IU | Vitamin C: 0.5mg | Calcium: 2mg | Iron: 0.1mg

DESSERT

Low Fodmap Salted Caramel Banana Cake

Serving size: 14 Prep Time: 20 mins
Total Time: 20 mins

INGREDIENTS

Cake & Sauce:

- Two 8-inch (20 cm) Buttermilk Banana Cake rounds, cooked and chilled
- 1/3 cup (75 ml) + ¼ cup (60 ml) Salted Caramel Sauce, split for both Frosting and Decor
- Frosting:
- 1/2 cup (1 stick; 113 g) unsalted butter, softened
- 2 1/4 cups (202 g) confectioners' sugar
- 1/2 teaspoon vanilla extract
- Décor:
- 1 firm banana
- 12 pecan halves, toasted if you prefer
- Semisweet chocolate shavings optional

INSTRUCTIONS

1. For the Frosting: Cream the butter with an electric mixer on high speed until smooth and creamy. Add approximately half of the confectioners' sugar and mix until blended. Beat in the ⅓ cup (75 ml) of the Salted Caramel Sauce and vanilla, then add remaining confectioners' sugar and continue beating until extremely smooth and creamy and everything is incorporated very well.

2. To Cake Assembly & Décor: Place one cake layer on the display plate and spread approximately half of the frosting on top, going all the way to the edge. (I used a pastry bag and a 1/2-inch/12 mm round tip, but you can simply spread it on with an offset spatula). Place the second cake layer on top. Spread the remaining frosting over the top, concentrating on the middle of the cake; no need to go to the edge.

3. Right before serving, peel and slice the banana and arrange the pieces here and there, nestling within the icing. Use the photographs for inspiration. Tuck the pecans around the banana slices. Make sure the remaining ¼ cup (60 ml) of Salted Caramel Sauce is fluid,

but not hot and sprinkle over the cake, allowing it to trickle down the edges. Sprinkle the chocolate shavings on top, if using, and serve ideally within the hour.

NUTRITION

Calories: 316 kcal | Carbohydrates: 53g | Protein: 2g | Fat: 11g | Cholesterol: 3mg | Sodium: 1mg | Fiber: 1g | Sugar: 41g | Vitamin A: 25 IU | Vitamin C: 0.1mg | Calcium: 1mg

---

Pumpkin Cheesecake With Gingersnap Crust

Serving size: 18 Prep Time: 20 mins
Cook Time: 1 hour 30 mins Total Time: 1 hour 50
mins

INGREDIENTS

Crust:

- 1, 7- ounce bag Tate's Bake Shop Gluten-Free Ginger Zinger Cookies or enough low-FODMAP cookie crumbs of choice to equal 1 ⅓ to 1 ½ cups 315 ml to 360 ml
- 2 tablespoons unsalted butter melted
- Cheesecake:

- 4, 8- ounce (227 g) packages Green Valley Lactose Free Cream Cheese, at room temperature
- 3/4 cup (149 g) sugar
- 1 cup (269 g) canned pumpkin purée
- 1 teaspoon cinnamon
- ½ teaspoon ground ginger
- ¼ teaspoon ground cloves
- ¼ teaspoon freshly grated nutmeg
- 1/2 teaspoon vanilla extract
- 5 big eggs at room temperature, whisked very thoroughly in a bowl
- 1 cup (227 g) Green Valley Lactose Free Sour Cream, at room temperature

INSTRUCTIONS

For the Crust:

1. Position rack in middle of oven. Preheat the oven to 375°F/190°C. Coat the interior of a 9-inch (23 cm) springform pan with nonstick spray. Double wrap the outside of the pan with extra-wide aluminum foil, bringing the foil all the way up and around the edges of the pan to the top edge; set aside.
2. Grind the cookies to a fine crumb in a food processor equipped with a metal blade.

Alternatively, put in a hefty zip top bag and crush firmly with a rolling pin. Use a rolling and a smashing action to get the job done. Stir in melted butter to evenly moist crumbs. Press crust mixture firmly into an equal layer on the bottom of the prepared pan.

3. Bake for approximately 10 to 12 minutes or until light golden brown. You want the cookies to dry out a little. Remove crust from oven and lay aside on rack. Turn the oven down 325°F/165°F.

For the Cheesecake:

1. Meanwhile, make the cheesecake batter. Lactose-free cream cheese functions differently from conventional cream cheese so please follow our technique: put one container of cream cheese in a mixing dish and combine on low speed with an electric mixer until creamy and smooth. Add sugar, pumpkin purée, spices and vanilla and combine very briefly on low speed. Pour in eggs a little bit at a time, mixing just enough to combine and no more. Mixture could be quite liquid at this stage; that's alright. Add remaining cream cheese and beat just until incorporated, approximately 30 seconds to 1

minute. If the cream cheese is resisting being mixed with the first mixture, use a big balloon whisk and incorporate by hand using a folding movement. Make sure the mixture is properly blended but do not over mix. Gently whisk in sour cream by hand. Scrape cheesecake batter over crust.

2. Place aluminum foil coated pan in a large roasting pan. Add extremely hot tap water to the roasting pan to come up the edges of the springform pan approximately 1-inch (2.5 cm). Bake for 1 hour to 1 hour and 5 minutes. Cake should be set at the edges and slightly giggly in the middle. Turn the oven off, leaving the cake in the oven for 15 minutes longer.

3. Remove from the oven. Dip the tip of a small paring knife in warm water and use it to run over the top edge of the cake (moving down about ½ inch/12 mm) to loosen it from the pan; this will prevent the sides from coming away from the pan, which may produce cracks. Remove cake pan and remove foil. Refrigerate overnight or up to 48 hours. Dip a tiny icing spatula in warm water, shake dry, and run all the way around the outside border

of the cake going all the way down to the bottom to release the cake from the pan. Release springform, remove and arrange cake on a presentation dish.

NUTRITION

Calories: 357 kcal | Carbohydrates: 25g | Protein: 4g | Fat: 27g | Saturated Fat: 1g | Sodium: 17mg | Fiber: 1g | Sugar: 17g | Vitamin A: 220IU | Calcium: 10mg

---

Rhubarb Pie With Lattice Crust

Serving size: 10 Prep Time: 30 mins
Cook Time: 30 mins Total Time: 1 hour

INGREDIENTS

- 1 batch All-Butter Pie Crust dough ready to roll
- Filling:
- 1 1/2 pounds (680 g) rhubarb, cut into ½-inch (12 mm) pieces
- 1 1/3 cups (263 g) sugar
- 3 tablespoons cornstarch
- 1/8 teaspoon cinnamon
- 1 tablespoon unsalted butter

- Topping:
- 2 tablespoons lactose-free whole milk
- 2 tablespoons sugar

INSTRUCTIONS

1. Have our double pie crust recipe prepared, refrigerated and ready to roll out. For the Filling: Position rack in the lowest third of your oven. Preheat to 425° F/220°C. Coat a 9-inch (23 cm), ovenproof glass pie dish with nonstick spray; leave aside.

2. Stir together the rhubarb, 1 ⅓ cups (263 g) sugar, cornstarch and cinnamon in a bowl. Allow to rest for 15 minutes until fluids begin to exude while the oven preheats.

3. Roll out 1 dough disc on a gently floured surface to a 12-inch (30.5 cm) circle. Transfer to a pie dish. Trim edges to 1 inch (2.5 cm) all around. Fold extra crust under itself toward the outside of the pan; crimp the edge.

4. Stir filling together with any juices that have seeped and pour into the crust. Dot the surface evenly with little chunks of butter.

5. Roll out a second dough disc to a 12-inch (30.5 cm) circle and cut into 1-inch-wide (2.5 cm) strips using either a straight edge or

fluted pastry wheel. Brush the crimped edge gently with water. Weave a lattice crust on top of the filling. Trim the lattice strips to fit the plate and press hard to seal along the crimped edge. Brush the lattice with milk and sprinkle it with sugar.

6. Bake for 15 minutes; turn the oven down to 375° F/190° C and continue baking until the crust is golden brown and the filling is bubbling, approximately 30 to 35 minutes longer. Cool on rack for at least 2 hours to enable fluids to thicken. Serve heated or at room temperature. Store at room temperature overnight, lightly wrapped with foil, if preferred.

NUTRITION
Calories: 322 kcal | Carbohydrates: 55g | Protein: 3g | Fat: 11g | Cholesterol: 21mg | Sodium: 69mg | Fiber: 1g | Sugar: 35g | Vitamin A: 30IU | Calcium: 3mg | Iron: 0.1mg

Strawberry Shortcakes With Buttermilk Biscuits

Serving size: 8 Prep Time: 20 mins
Cook Time:12 mins Total Time: 32 mins

INGREDIENTS
Biscuits:

- 1/2 cup (120 ml) lactose-free whole milk, cooled
- 11/2 tablespoons lemon juice, ideally freshly squeezed
- 1 big egg, cooled
- 1 1/2 cups (218 g) low FODMAP gluten free all-purpose flour, such as Bob's Red Mill Gluten Free 1 to 1 Baking Flour
- 3 tablespoons sugar
- 1 tablespoon baking powder; use gluten-free if following a gluten-free diet
- 1/2 teaspoon baking soda
- 1/2 teaspoon salt
- 1/2 cup (1 stick; 113 g) unsalted butter, cold, cut into pieces

Strawberry Filling:

- 1 quart (590 g) strawberries, ideally small to medium sized, split

- 1/4 cup (50 g) sugar, split
- 1 1/2 tablespoons lemon juice, ideally freshly squeezed
- Whipped Cream Topping:
- 1 1/2 cups (360 ml) heavy cream, ideally lactose-free, cooled
- 2 tablespoons sugar

INSTRUCTIONS

For the Shortcakes:

1. Position rack in middle of oven. Preheat the oven to 425°F/220°C. Line a baking sheet pan with parchment paper; put aside.
2. In a small dish mix the milk and lemon juice and leave it to rest for 5 minutes to thicken, then whisk in egg; put aside.
3. In a large mixing basin, whisk together the flour, sugar, baking powder, baking soda and salt to aerate and incorporate. Cut in the butter with a pastry blender or two knives until the butter varies in size from big flat raisins to little peas. (You can also do this in a stand mixer with the flat paddle attachment, pulsing on and off).
4. Add the wet mixture to the dry ingredients and gently blend together by swirling with a

wooden spoon just until incorporated. Very carefully pat out the dough on a very lightly floured board to a 7 by 4 inch (17 cm by 10 cm) rectangle. Cut into 8 equal pieces then gently use your hands to mold each piece into a round biscuit approximately ¾ to 1 inch (2 cm to 2.5 cm) thick. Arrange the biscuits on the prepared pan, evenly spaced apart.

5. Bake for approximately 8 to 12 minutes or until tops and bottoms are slightly tinged with color and the biscuit is cooked all the way through. Place the pan on a cooling rack until the biscuits are totally cold, at which time they are ready to use. Alternatively, keep at room temperature for up to 8 hours, lightly covered in foil.

For the Filling:

1. Remove the stems from the strawberries and discard. Roughly chop half of them and mix with 3 tablespoons of the sugar in a saucepan. Stir well to incorporate and simmer over medium heat, stirring regularly, until the fruit is boiling and juicy, approximately 5 minutes. The juices should deepen and concentrate. Cool fully. Halve or quarter the remaining berries (depending on size, you could even

want to slice them; they should be bite size).
Toss these fresh berries with the remaining
sugar and the lemon juice in a dish and leave
to rest, tossing regularly, until the juices seep
and the sugar melts, approximately 15
minutes. Fold the two berry mixtures
together. Use immediately or refrigerate for
up to 3 hours in an airtight container.

2. For the Assembly: Right before serving,
    combine the cream and sugar for the topping
    and beat with an electric mixer on high speed
    just until mixture is noticeably thickened,
    then drop the speed and continue to whisk
    just until very soft peaks form. Do not
    over-whip or you will lose the smooth
    texture.

3. Pry the shortcakes in half horizontally with a
    fork. Place the bottom half, cut side up, on 8
    dessert plates or in shallow basins. Spoon
    over a substantial number of strawberries and
    juice, top with a hefty dollop of cream, then
    crown with the top of the biscuit. Allow it to
    settle for around 5 minutes for the fluids to
    enter the biscuit. Serve immediately.

NUTRITION

Calories: 370 kcal | Carbohydrates: 27g | Protein: 3g | Fat: 29g | Saturated Fat: 10g | Cholesterol: 87 mg | Sodium: 374 mg | Potassium: 224mg | Fiber: 2g | Sugar: 22g | Vitamin A: 705IU | Vitamin C: 71.5mg | Calcium: 52mg | Iron: 0.6mg

---

Almond Milk Chocolate Pudding

Serving size: 8 Prep Time: 10 mins
Cook Time: 8 mins Total Time: 18 mins

INGREDIENTS

- 1/3 cup (28 g) sifting natural cocoa
- 1/3 cup (65 g) sugar
- 2 tablespoons cornstarch
- Pinch salt
- 2 cups (480 ml) unsweetened almond milk, such as Almond Breeze Unsweetened
- 2 ounces (55 g) semisweet or bittersweet chocolate, coarsely chopped, ideally about 55% to 60% (55% to 61%)
- 1 teaspoon vanilla extract
- Coconut Whipped Cream, optional
- Chocolate shavings

INSTRUCTIONS

1. Have 8 ramekins, goblets or glasses ready to accept the pudding.

2. Whisk together the cocoa, sugar, cornstarch and salt in a medium-sized pot. Slowly whisk in approximately half of the almond milk until smooth, then whisk in remaining almond milk.

3. Bring to a simmer over low-medium heat, (may take around 3 to 5 minutes), then simmer for 1 minute, whisking constantly until it appears thickened and you can see faint whisk marks. Add chocolate and whisk constantly for approximately 1 minute longer until chocolate melts and the pudding is thick and creamy. The pudding should be thick enough to leave distinct whisk marks on the surface. Remove from heat, whisk in vanilla, then quickly pour into ready plates or goblets.

4. Now, you have an option. You presumably expected that the pudding had to cool down and then even be chilled. So you may serve warm or chill till about room temperature, then refrigerate at least 2 hours or overnight until set. Serve chilled with the optional

whipped coconut cream topping. A very light shaving of chocolate is a wonderful addition. If you add this decorative touch, go extremely mild on the chocolate to keep FODMAPs in control.

NUTRITION

Calories: 96 kcal | Carbohydrates: 18g | Protein: 1g | Fat: 2g | Sodium: 1mg | Fiber: 1g | Sugar: 13g

---

Low Fodmap Chocolate Shell

Servings size: 6 Prep Time: 5 mins
Total Time: 5 mins

INGREDIENTS

- 6 ounces (170 g) semisweet chocolate, coarsely chopped, between 47% and 55% cacao mass
- 2 tbsp refined coconut oil

INSTRUCTIONS

1. Melt the chocolate and coconut oil together in a microwave safe dish in the microwave on half power or on top of a double boiler. When

three-quarters of their way melted, remove from fire and carefully whisk until chocolate is melted and mixture is smooth. Allow to cool a little bit before drizzling over ice cream.

2. I prefer to cook this just before I need it. You may chill in an airtight jar and reheat before using

NUTRITION

Calories: 204 kcal | Carbohydrates: 15g | Protein: 2g | Fat: 16g | Saturated Fat: 6g | Cholesterol: 2mg | Sodium: 3mg | Potassium: 161mg | Fiber: 2g | Sugar: 10g | Vitamin A: 15IU | Calcium: 18mg | Iron: 1.8mg

---

Low Fodmap Apple Strudel

Servings size: 20 Prep Time: 15 mins
Cook Time: 15 mins Total Time: 30 mins

INGREDIENTS

- 3 Pink Lady apples, cored, peeled and coarsely diced to yield 300 g of chopped apple

- 1/4 cup (54 g) firmly packed light brown sugar
- 3 tablespoons chopped raisins
- 3 tablespoons finely chopped walnuts
- 2 teaspoons cornstarch
- 1 1/2 teaspoons cinnamon
- 1 teaspoon lemon zest
- 8 sheets of filo dough
- 1/4 cup (57 g) unsalted butter, melted
- 3 tablespoons low FODMAP, gluten-free panko

INSTRUCTIONS

1. Position rack in center of oven. Preheat the oven to 350°F/180°C. Line a rimmed half-sheet pan with parchment paper; put aside.

2. Stir the finely chopped apples, brown sugar, raisins, walnuts, cornstarch, cinnamon and lemon zest together in a small bowl until thoroughly blended.

3. Lay one sheet of filo on your work area horizontally (I prefer to do this on a clean piece of parchment paper) and brush with butter. Add another sheet, more butter and repeat until you have used 4 sheets of filo

altogether, concluding with brushing butter on top. Sprinkle half of the panko all over (do this by eye) then put half of the apple filling in a "log" form down the long end near you. Firmly roll the log up away from you, folding in the sides as you reach the final half. Place seam side down on the prepared pan. Repeat with remaining filo and filling. You should have two logs, spread equally apart on your baking pan. Brush tops with melted butter. (You may hold the strudel at this stage, wrapped with plastic wrap and refrigerated, up to overnight. Some people have even had luck with freezing. Take care to bring it to room temperature before baking.)

4. Bake for approximately 15 minutes or until golden brown and crispy. Allow to cool on pans placed on racks for at least 5 minutes. Use a sharp serrated knife to cut crosswise into 10 pieces each. Serve heated or at room temperature. These are best served the day they are cooked.

NUTRITION

Calories: 75 kcal | Carbohydrates: 10g | Protein: 1g | Fat: 3g | Saturated Fat: 1g | Sodium: 1mg | Fiber: 1g | Sugar: 5g | Vitamin C: 0.2mg | Calcium: 2mg

---

Low Fodmap Grape & Apple Crisp

Servings size: 16 Prep Time: 10 mins
Cook Time: 45 mins Total Time: 55 mins

INGREDIENTS

- Grape & Apple Filling:
- 3 cups (450 g) seedless red grapes, halved
- 2 cups (240 g) chopped peeled Pink Lady apples
- Crisp Topping:
- 6 tablespoons (85 g) unsalted butter
- 3/4 cup (160 g) firmly packed light brown sugar
- 1/2 cup (73 g) + 1 tablespoon low FODMAP gluten-free flour, such as Bob's Red Mill Gluten Free 1 to 1 Baking Flour
- 1/2 cup (50 g) + 1 tablespoon old-fashioned rolled oats (not instant or quick oats); use gluten-free if following a gluten-free diet

- Heaping ¼ teaspoon cinnamon
- Heaping ⅛ teaspoon salt

INSTRUCTIONS

1. Preheat the oven to 375°F/190°C. Coat a 9-inch (23 cm) pie pan with nonstick spray; put aside.

2. Place the grapes and apples into the pie pan and toss together to blend

3. For the Crisp Topping: Melt the butter in a medium-size microwave-safe mixing dish in the microwave on low. (Or melt the butter in a small pot on your stove top, if you want, then transfer to a medium-size mixing bowl.) Whisk in the brown sugar, then whisk in the flour, oats, cinnamon, and salt until thoroughly incorporated. Use your hands to help make clumps then spread them evenly over the fruit resting in the pie pan.

4. Bake for approximately 40 to 45 minutes or until the filling is bubbling and the topping is golden brown. Let sit for 5 minutes before serving. The Low FODMAP Grape & Apple Crisp may be served warm, at room temperature, or re-warmed after chilling and is best the day it is cooked. You may keep it

at room temperature gently wrapped with foil overnight but the topping will lose a little of its crispness.

NUTRITION

Calories: 124 kcal | Carbohydrates: 21g | Protein: 1g | Fat: 4g | Sodium: 9mg | Fiber: 1g | Sugar: 15g

SEAFOOD RECIPES

Grilled Salmon with Lemon Herb Sauce

Servings: 4 Prep time: 15 minutes
Cooking time: 10 minutes

INGREDIENTS

- 4 salmon filets - 2 teaspoons olive oil
- Salt and pepper to taste
- For the Lemon Herb Sauce:
- 1/4 cup fresh parsley, chopped
- 1/4 cup fresh chives, chopped
- Zest and juice of 1 lemon
- 2 tablespoons olive oil
- Salt and pepper to taste

INSTRUCTIONS

1. Preheat the grill to medium-high heat.
2. Season the salmon filets with olive oil, salt, and pepper.
3. Place the salmon filets on the grill and cook for approximately 4-5 minutes each side, or until cooked through.
4. In a separate bowl, whisk together the parsley, chives, lemon zest, lemon juice, olive

oil, salt, and pepper to create the Lemon Herb Sauce.

5. Serve the cooked salmon with the Lemon Herb Sauce poured on top.

NUTRITION

Calories: 300
Protein: 25g - Carbohydrates: 2g
Fat: 20g, Fiber: 1g

Shrimp Stir-Fry with Vegetables

Servings: 4 Prep time: 20 mins
Cooking time: 15 mins

INGREDIENTS

- pound shrimp, peeled and deveined - 2 teaspoons garlic-infused olive oil
- 1 red bell pepper, sliced - 1 zucchini, sliced - 1 carrot, julienned - 1 cup bok choy, chopped - 2 tablespoons low-sodium soy sauce
- Salt and pepper to taste

INSTRUCTIONS

1. Heat the garlic-infused olive oil in a large pan over medium heat.
2. Add the shrimp and heat for approximately 2-3 minutes on each side until pink and cooked through. Remove from the skillet and put aside.
3. In the same pan, add the red bell pepper, zucchini, carrot, and bok choy. Cook for approximately 5-7 minutes until veggies are tender-crisp.
4. Add the cooked shrimp back to the skillet.
5. Drizzle with low-sodium soy sauce and season with salt and pepper. Stir well to mix.
6. Serve the shrimp stir-fry hot.

NUTRITION

Calories: 200
Protein: 20g - Carbohydrates: 8g
Fat: 10g, Fiber: 3g

Grilled Shrimp Skewers with Lemon Garlic Marinade

Servings: 4   Prep time: 20 mins

Cooking time: 6 mins

INGREDIENTS

- 1 pound big shrimp, peeled and deveined - 2 teaspoons garlic-infused olive oil
- Zest and juice of 1 lemon
- 2 tablespoons fresh parsley, chopped - Salt & pepper to taste

INSTRUCTIONS

1. In a bowl, mix the garlic-infused olive oil, lemon zest, lemon juice, parsley, salt, and pepper to prepare the marinade.
2. Add the shrimp to the marinade and let it rest for approximately 15-20 minutes.
3. Thread the marinated shrimp on skewers.
4. Preheat the grill to medium-high heat and grill the shrimp skewers for approximately 2-3 minutes each side until cooked through.
5. Serve the grilled shrimp skewers hot.

NUTRITION

Calories: 150

Protein: 20g - Carbohydrates: 2g

Fat: 7g, Fiber: 0g

Baked Cod with Herb Crust

Servings: 4 Prep time: 10 mis
Cooking time: 15 mins

INGREDIENTS

- 4 cod filets - 2 tablespoons fresh parsley, chopped - 2 tablespoons fresh chives, chopped
- Zest of 1 lemon - 2 tablespoons olive oil - Salt and pepper to taste

INSTRUCTION

1. Preheat the oven to 400°F (200°C).
2. Season the fish filets with salt and pepper and set them on a baking sheet.
3. In a bowl, mix together the parsley, chives, lemon zest, olive oil, salt, and pepper to form the herb crust.
4. Spread the herb crust mixture equally over the top of each fish filet.
5. Bake in the preheated oven for around 12-15 minutes or until the fish is cooked through.
6. Serve the baked cod hot.

NUTRITION

Calories: 180
Protein: 25g - Carbohydrates: 1g
Fat: 8g, Fiber: 0g

Lemon Butter Shrimp Stir-Fry

Serving Size: 4
Preparation Time: 15 mins

INGREDIENTS

- 1 pound shrimp, peeled and deveined
- 3 tablespoons unsalted butter
- 2 teaspoons lemon juice
- 1 teaspoon garlic-infused oil
- 1/2 teaspoon paprika
- Salt and pepper to taste

INSTRUCTIONS

1. Heat butter and garlic-infused oil in a pan over medium-high heat.
2. Add shrimp to the pan and cook until pink and opaque.
3. Stir in lemon juice and paprika. Season with salt and pepper.

4. Cook for a further 2-3 minutes, ensuring shrimp are thoroughly cooked.
5. Serve the shrimp stir-fry warm.

NUTRITION

Calories: 240
Protein: 26g, Fat: 14g
Carbohydrates: 1g, Fiber: 0g

Grilled Swordfish with Cilantro Lime Marinade

Serving Size: 4 Prep Time: 30 mins (including marinating time)

INGREDIENTS

- 4 swordfish steaks
- 3 tablespoons olive oil
- 2 tablespoons fresh cilantro, chopped Zest and juice of 1 lime
- 1 teaspoon ground cumin
- Salt and pepper to taste

INSTRUCTIONS

1. Preheat the grill to medium-high heat.

2. In a bowl, combine olive oil, chopped cilantro, lime zest, lime juice, cumin, salt, and pepper.
3. Brush the swordfish steaks with the marinade.
4. Grill the swordfish for 4-5 minutes each side or until cooked through.
5. Serve the grilled swordfish with an additional sprinkle of the cilantro lime marinade.

NUTRITION

Calories: 300
Protein: 30g, Fat: 18g
Carbohydrates: 1g
Fiber: 0.5g

Low FODMAP Cajun Shrimp Skewers

Serving Size: 4
Preparation Time: 20 minutes (including skewering time)

INGREDIENTS
- 1 pound big shrimp, peeled and deveined
- 2 tablespoons olive oil

- 1 teaspoon paprika
- 1/2 teaspoon dried oregano
- 1/2 teaspoon ground cayenne pepper (adjust to taste)
- Salt and pepper to taste
- Lemon wedges for serving

INSTRUCTIONS

1. Preheat the grill or grill pan to medium-high heat.
2. In a bowl, add olive oil, paprika, oregano, cayenne pepper, salt, and pepper.
3. Thread shrimp on skewers and brush with the Cajun spice mixture.
4. Grill the shrimp skewers for 2-3 minutes each side or until they are cooked through.
5. Serve the Cajun shrimp skewers with lemon wedges.

NUTRITION

Calories: 220
Protein: 25g, Fat: 12g
Carbohydrates: 2g, Fiber: 0.5g

Garlic Lemon Butter Scallops

Serving Size: 4
Preparation Time: 15 mins

INGREDIENTS

- 1 pound scallops, patted dry
- 3 tablespoons unsalted butter
- 3 cloves garlic, minced
- 1 tablespoon fresh lemon juice
- 1 teaspoon fresh parsley, chopped
- Salt and pepper to taste

INSTRUCTIONS

1. Heat butter in a pan over medium-high heat.
2. Add minced garlic and sauté until fragrant.
3. Add scallops to the skillet and cook for 2-3 minutes each side until golden brown.
4. Stir in lemon juice, chopped parsley, salt, and pepper.
5. Cook for a further minute, ensuring scallops are thoroughly cooked.
6. Serve the garlic lemon butter scallops warm.

NUTRITION

Calories: 180

Protein: 20g, Fat: 10g
Carbohydrates: 3g, Fiber: 0g

Herb-Crusted Baked Tilapia

Serving Size: 4
Prep Time: 20 mins

INGREDIENTS

- 4 tilapia filets
- 2 tablespoons olive oil
- 2 tablespoons fresh parsley, chopped 1 tablespoon fresh chives, chopped 1 teaspoon dried dill
- 1 teaspoon lemon zest
- Salt and pepper to taste

INSTRUCTIONS

1. Preheat the oven to 400°F (200°C).
2. Place tilapia filets on a baking sheet.
3. In a bowl, combine olive oil, chopped parsley, chives, dill, lemon zest, salt, and pepper.
4. Spread the herb mixture over the tilapia filets.

5. Bake for 12-15 minutes or until the fish readily flakes with a fork.
6. Serve the herb-crusted tilapia warm.

NUTRITION
Calories: 150
Protein: 25g, Fat: 6g
Carbohydrates: 1g, Fiber: 0g

Lemon Herb Grilled Prawns

Serving. Size: 4
Prep Time: 25 mins (including skewering time)

INGREDIENTS
- 1 pound big prawns, peeled and deveined 3 tablespoons olive oil
- 2 tablespoons fresh basil, chopped
- 1 tablespoon fresh mint, chopped Zest and juice of 1 lemon
- Salt and pepper to taste

INSTRUCTIONS

1. In a bowl, combine olive oil, chopped basil, mint, lemon zest, lemon juice, salt, and pepper.
2. Thread prawns on skewers and brush with the herb and lemon mixture.
3. Preheat the grill to medium-high heat.
4. Grill the prawn skewers for 2-3 minutes each side until they are cooked through.
5. Serve the lemon herb grilled prawns warm.

NUTRITION

Calories: 230
Protein: 24g, Fat: 14g
Carbohydrates: 2g, Fiber: 0.5g

Seared Tuna Steaks with Sesame Crust

Serving Size: 4 Prep Time: 20 mins

INGREDIENTS

- 4 tuna steaks
- 2 teaspoons sesame seeds
- 2 tablespoons soy sauce (check for FODMAP-friendly components)

- 1 tablespoon sesame oil
- 1 tablespoon green onion tops, finely chopped
- 1 teaspoon grated ginger
- 1 teaspoon rice vinegar

INSTRUCTIONS

1. Rub tuna steaks with sesame seeds, pressing them into the surface.
2. In a bowl, mix together soy sauce, sesame oil, green onion tops, ginger, and rice vinegar.
3. Heat a pan over high heat and sear tuna steaks for 1-2 minutes each side for a rare to medium-rare cook.
4. Slice the tuna steaks and sprinkle with the soy-ginger sauce.

NUTRITION

Calories: 260
Protein: 30g, Fat: 13g
Carbohydrates: 3g, Fiber: 0.5g

Garlic Butter Baked Lobster Tails

Serving Size: 4

Prep Time: 25 mins

INGREDIENTS

- 4 lobster tails, divided in half
- 1/2 cup unsalted butter, melted 4 cloves garlic, minced 2 tablespoons fresh parsley, chopped
- Salt and pepper to taste
- Lemon wedges for serving

INSTRUCTIONS

1. Preheat the oven to 425°F (220°C).
2. Arrange lobster tails on a baking sheet.
3. In a bowl, combine melted butter, minced garlic, chopped parsley, salt, and pepper.
4. Brush the garlic butter mixture over the lobster tails.
5. Bake for 12-15 minutes or until the lobster flesh is opaque.
6. Serve the garlic butter roasted lobster tails with lemon wedges.

NUTRITION

Calories: 250
Protein: 28g, Fat: 15g
Carbohydrates: 1g, Fiber: 0g

Pesto Grilled Shrimp Skewers

Serving Size: 4
Prep Time: 20 mins (plus marinating time)

INGREDIENTS

- 1 pound big shrimp, peeled and deveined
- 1/2 cup Low FODMAP basil pesto (store-bought or homemade)
- 2 tablespoons olive oil
- 1 tablespoon lemon juice
- Salt and pepper to taste

INSTRUCTIONS

1. In a bowl, add shrimp, basil pesto, olive oil, lemon juice, salt, and pepper. Let it marinade for at least 15 minutes.
2. Thread shrimp on skewers.
3. Preheat the grill to medium-high heat.
4. Grill the shrimp skewers for 2-3 minutes each side or until they are cooked through.
5. Serve the pesto grilled shrimp skewers warm.

NUTRITION
Calories: 280
Protein: 26g, Fat: 18g
Carbohydrates: 3g, Fiber: 0.5g

VEGETABLE RECIPES

Roasted Carrots And Zucchini

Servings size: 4 Prep Time: 10 mins

INGREDIENT

- Carrots, peeled and sliced into sticks, four medium-sized carrots
- Two zucchinis of medium size, cut, and two tablespoons of olive oil
- To taste, season with salt and pepper
- Herbs that are fresh (optional)

INSTRUCTIONS

1. Preheat the oven to 400°F (200°C).
2. The carrots and zucchini should be tossed with olive oil, salt and pepper in a large basin after being prepared.
3. Spread the veggies in a single layer on a baking sheet.
4. Roast in the oven for 20-25 minutes or until veggies are soft and slightly browned.
5. Sprinkle with fresh herbs before serving.

NUTRITION

120 calories total

Carbohydrates: 10g, Fat: 8g

Protein: 2g, Fiber: 3g

Grilled Eggplant with Tomato Salsa

Servings: 2 Prep time: 15 mins

INGREDIENT

- 1 medium eggplant, cut
- 1 tablespoon olive oil
- To taste, season with salt and pepper
- For the salsa:
- 1 big tomato, chopped
- 1/4 cup chopped fresh parsley
- 1 tablespoon lemon juice
- To taste, season with salt and pepper

INSTRUCTIONS

1. Preheat the grill to medium-high heat.
2. Brush the eggplant slices with olive oil and season with salt and pepper.
3. Grill the eggplant slices for approximately 5 minutes each side or until cooked.

4. In a bowl, add the chopped tomato, parsley, lemon juice, salt, and pepper to create the salsa.
5. Serve the grilled eggplant topped with the tomato salsa.

NUTRITION
Calories: 150
Carbohydrates: 15g, Fat: 9g
Protein: 3g, Fiber: 7g

Quinoa Stuffed Bell Peppers

Servings: 4 Prep Time: 30 mins

INGREDIENTS
- 4 bell peppers, tops removed and seeds removed
- 1 cup quinoa, cooked
- 1 can (15 oz) black beans, washed and drained
- 1 cup corn kernels
- 1/2 cup chopped tomatoes
- 1 teaspoon cumin
- 1 teaspoon chili powder

- To taste, season with salt and pepper
- Optional toppings: avocado slices, cilantro, lime wedges

INSTRUCTIONS

1. Preheat the oven to 375°F (190°C).
2. In a large bowl, mix together the cooked quinoa, black beans, corn, chopped tomatoes, cumin, chili powder, salt, and pepper.
3. Stuff each bell pepper with the quinoa mixture and set them in a baking dish.
4. Cover the dish with aluminum foil and bake for 25-30 minutes or until the peppers are cooked.
5. Serve the filled bell peppers with optional toppings like avocado slices, cilantro, and lime wedges.

NUTRITION

Calories: 300
Carbohydrates: 55g
Fat: 4g Protein: 12g, Fiber: 11g

Lemon Herb Grilled Chicken

Servings: 4 Prep Time: 20 mins

INGREDIENTS

- 4 boneless, skinless chicken breasts
- Zest and juice of 1 lemon
- 2 tablespoons olive oil
- 2 cloves garlic, minced
- 1 teaspoon dried oregano
- To taste, season with salt and pepper

INSTRUCTIONS

1. In a bowl, mix together the lemon zest, lemon juice, olive oil, minced garlic, oregano, salt, and pepper.
2. Place the chicken breasts in a resealable plastic bag and pour the marinade over them. Seal the bag and chill for at least 30 minutes.
3. Preheat the grill to medium-high heat.
4. Grill the chicken breasts for approximately 6-7 minutes each side or until cooked through.
5. Let the chicken rest for a few minutes before serving.

NUTRITION
Calories: 200
Carbohydrates: 2g, Fat: 9g
Protein: 28g, Fiber: 0g

Greek Salad

Servings: 4 Prep Time: 15 mins

INGREDIENTS
- 2 big cucumbers, diced 4 medium tomatoes, diced
- 1/2 red onion, finely sliced
- 1/2 cup Kalamata olives
- 1/2 cup crumbled feta cheese
- 2 tablespoons olive oil
- 1 tablespoon red wine vinegar
- 1 teaspoon dried oregano
- To taste, season with salt and pepper

INSTRUCTIONS
1. In a large bowl, mix the cucumbers, tomatoes, red onion, Kalamata olives, and feta cheese.

2. In a small bowl, mix together the olive oil, red wine vinegar, dried oregano, salt, and pepper.
3. Pour the dressing over the salad and toss to mix.
4. Serve the Greek salad cold as a pleasant side dish.

A SUGAR SUGAR
Calories: 180
Carbohydrates: 12g
Fat: 14g, Protein: 5g, Fiber: 3g

Baked Salmon with Dill Sauce

Servings: 4 Prep Time: 25 mins

INGREDIENTS
- 4 salmon filets
- 1 tablespoon olive oil
- To taste, season with salt and pepper
- 1/4 cup plain lactose-free yogurt
- 1 tablespoon fresh dill, chopped
- 1 teaspoon lemon juice
- 1 clove garlic, minced

INSTRUCTIONS

1. Preheat the oven to 400°F (200°C).
2. Place the salmon filets on a baking pan lined with parchment paper.
3. Drizzle the salmon filets with olive oil and season with salt and pepper.
4. Bake the fish for around 15-20 minutes or until cooked through.
5. In a separate bowl, whisk together the yogurt, fresh dill, lemon juice, and chopped garlic to form the sauce.
6. Serve the cooked salmon with the dill sauce on top.

NUTRITION

Calories: 250
Carbohydrates: 2g, Fat: 15g
Protein: 25g, Fiber: 0g

Turkey and Vegetable Stir-Fry

Servings: 4 Prep Time: 20 mins

INGREDIENTS

- 1 pound ground turkey
- 2 cups mixed veggies (bell peppers, zucchini, carrots)
- 2 teaspoons low-sodium soy sauce
- 1 tablespoon sesame oil
- 1 teaspoon ginger, minced
- 1 clove garlic, minced
- To taste, season with salt and pepper

INSTRUCTIONS

- In a large pan, saute the ground turkey over medium heat until browned.
- Add the mixed veggies, ginger, and garlic to the pan and stir-fry for a few minutes until the vegetables are soft.
- Add the soy sauce, sesame oil, salt, and pepper to the skillet and combine thoroughly.
- Continue cooking for another few minutes until everything is cooked through.
- Serve the turkey and veggie stir-fry hot.

NUTRITION

Calories: 280
Carbohydrates: 8g, Fat: 16g
Protein: 26g, Fiber: 2g

Quinoa Salad with Roasted Vegetables

Servings: 4 Prep Time: 30 mins

INGREDIENTS

- 1 cup quinoa, cooked
- 2 cups mixed roasted vegetables (bell peppers, eggplant, cherry tomatoes)
- 1/4 cup pine nuts
- 1/4 cup fresh basil, chopped
- 2 tablespoons olive oil
- 1 tablespoon balsamic vinegar
- To taste, season with salt and pepper

INSTRUCTIONS

1. In a large bowl, mix the cooked quinoa, roasted veggies, pine nuts, and fresh basil.
2. In a small bowl, mix together the olive oil, balsamic vinegar, salt, and pepper to create the dressing.
3. Pour the dressing over the quinoa salad and toss to mix.
4. Serve the quinoa salad at room temperature or chilled.

NUTRITION
Calories: 280
Carbohydrates: 30g, Fat: 14g
Protein: 8g, Fiber: 5g

Eggplant Parmesan

Servings: 4 Prep Time: 45 mins

INGREDIENT
- 1 big eggplant, cut into rounds
- 1 cup gluten-free breadcrumbs
- 1/2 cup grated Parmesan cheese
- 1 teaspoon dried oregano
- 1 teaspoon dried basil
- 1/2 teaspoon garlic powder
- To taste, season with salt and pepper
- 2 eggs, beaten
- 1 cup low-FODMAP marinara sauce
- 1 cup lactose-free mozzarella cheese, shredded
- Fresh basil leaves for garnish

INSTRUCTIONS

1. Preheat the oven to 375°F (190°C).
2. In a shallow dish, mix the breadcrumbs, Parmesan cheese, oregano, basil, garlic powder, salt, and pepper.
3. Dip each eggplant slice into the beaten eggs, then coat with the breadcrumb mixture.
4. Place the oiled eggplant slices on a baking sheet lined with parchment paper and bake for approximately 20 minutes until golden brown.
5. In a baking dish, put a layer of marinara sauce, then place the cooked eggplant slices on top.
6. Top the eggplant slices with the leftover marinara sauce and sprinkle with mozzarella cheese.
7. Bake for a further 15-20 minutes until the cheese is melted and bubbling.
8. Garnish with fresh basil leaves before serving.

NUTRITION

Calories: 280
Carbohydrates: 20g, Fat: 14g
Protein: 16g, Fiber: 5g

Roasted Brussels Sprouts with Bacon

Servings: 4 Prep time: 30 mins

INGREDIENT

1 pound Brussels sprouts, trimmed and halved 4 slices bacon, chopped 2 tablespoons olive oil
To taste, season with salt and pepper

INSTRUCTIONS

1. Preheat the oven to 400°F (200°C).
2. In a large dish, mix the Brussels sprouts with olive oil, salt, and pepper until thoroughly coated.
3. Spread the Brussels sprouts on a baking sheet in a single layer.
4. Scatter the diced bacon over the Brussels sprouts.
5. Roast in the oven for around 20-25 minutes until the Brussels sprouts are soft and caramelized.
6. Serve the roasted Brussels sprouts with bacon hot.

NUTRITION
Calories: 180
Carbohydrates: 10g, Fat: 14g
Protein: 6g, Fiber: 4g

REFRESHING DRINK & SMOOTHIE RECIPES

Low Fodmap Orange Carrot Juice

Servings size: 2 Prep Time:5 mins
Total Time: 5 mins

INGREDIENTS

- ½ cup (120 ml) freshly squeezed carrot juice
- ½ cup (120 ml) freshly squeezed orange juice
- Add-Ons: ¼ cup (60 ml) UHT unsweetened coconut milk
- 2 tablespoons low FODMAP whey protein isolate, such as Opportuniteas Grass-Fed Whey Protein Isolate Ice

INSTRUCTIONS

1. **Method #1:** Place carrot juice, orange juice, coconut milk, protein powder and ice in a blender and zap it until frothy, frosty and mixed. Serve immediately.
2. **Method #2:** Simply blend the carrot and orange juice, divide into two glasses and enjoy. Add ice if you like.

3. **Method #3:** Add the coconut milk to Version #1. I prefer to mix everything up in a jar, or you can use a blender. On the rocks or straight up.

NUTRITION

Calories: 79 kcal | Carbohydrates: 10g | Protein: 8g | Fat: 1g

---

Sparkling Ginger Cranberry Punch

Servings size: 7 Prep Time: 10 mins
Cook Time: 10 mins Total Time: 20 mins

INGREDIENTS

- Simple Syrup
- 1/4 cup (50 g) sugar
- 1/4 cup (60 ml) water
- Punch: 4 decaffeinated black tea bags
- 2 cups (480 ml) water
- 4 cups (960 ml) cranberry juice (see headnote), chilled 2 clementines, washed 1/2 lemon, washed 1/2 lime, washed 1 cup (150 g) red seedless grapes, split lengthwise, plus extra for garnish

INSTRUCTIONS

1. Make the Simple Syrup: Stir together the sugar and water in a small saucepan and bring to a boil over high heat. Boil for approximately 1 minute, turning the saucepan once or twice, until sugar dissolves. Set aside to cool.

2. Make the Punch: Place 4 tea bags in a heatproof vessel, such as a teapot or big Pyrex measuring cup. Bring 2 cups of water to a boil, pour over tea bags and let steep for 3 minutes. Remove and discard bags. Chill the brewed tea.

3. Combine the cold brewed tea with the cranberry juice in a big transparent pitcher. Slice the clementines, lemon and lime crosswise and add to the pitcher. Add the grapes. Sweetened to taste with the Simple Syrup, but remember that the ginger ale will provide some sweetness, too. Punch is ready to serve but is much nicer if you let fruit and drink to mingle for a few hours in the refrigerator.

NUTRITION

Calories: 118 kcal | Carbohydrates: 31g | Protein: 1g | Fat: 1g | Saturated Fat: 1g | Sodium: 7mg | Potassium: 152mg | Fiber: 1g | Sugar: 29g | Vitamin A: 60IU | Vitamin C: 27mg | Calcium: 21mg | Iron: 0.4mg

---

Low Fodmap Blueberry Limeade

Servings size 6. Prep Time: 10 mins
Total Time: 10 mins

INGREDIENTS

- 1 cup (160 g) blueberries
- 1/3 cup (65 g) sugar, plus more if required
- 4 cups (960 ml) water
- 6 tablespoons (90 ml) freshly squeezed lime juice
- Ice cubes
- Lime slices or wedges as garnish; optional

INSTRUCTIONS

1. Place blueberries in a non-reactive mixing basin, add sugar and mash very thoroughly with a potato masher. Allow it to settle for 5

minutes, then mash some more. Pour mixture into a fine-meshed strainer placed over a large pitcher, squeezing the mashed fruit as forcefully to extract as much juice as possible.

2. Whisk in the water and lime juice. Taste and adjust sweetness, if required. Pour over ice and add lime slices, if you prefer.

3. (Optional) Add one 6-gram amount of Regular Girl to each serving of Low FODMAP Blueberry Limeade and stir vigorously until dissolved. Your synbiotic drink is ready.

NUTRITION

Calories: 76 kcal | Carbohydrates: 19g | Sodium: 8mg | Potassium: 30mg | Sugar: 17g | Vitamin A: 20IU | Vitamin C: 3.8mg | Calcium: 7mg | Iron: 0.1mg

---

Low Fodmap Ginger Pomegranate Pear Sparkler

Serving size 1 Prep Time: 5 mins
Total Time: 5 mins

INGREDIENTS

- Ice cubes 6 ounces (180 ml) your sparkling ginger beverage of choice
- 5 gram piece of fresh pear
- 1 tablespoon pomegranate seeds

INSTRUCTIONS

1. Fill a big glass with ice cubes and pour in your sparkling ginger beverage. Slide that thin slice of pear down along the edge of the glass, sprinkle the pomegranate seeds on top and serve!
2. A straw or stirrer makes it even more festive.

NUTRITION

Calories: 77kcal | Carbohydrates: 19g | Protein: 1g | Fat: 1g | Saturated Fat: 1g | Sodium: 1mg | Potassium: 35mg | Fiber: 1g | Sugar: 17g | Vitamin C: 1.6mg

Maple Lime Low Fodmap Drink

Servings size: 2 Prep Time: 5 mins
Total Time: 5 mins

INGREDIENTS

- 3 1/2 cups (875 ml) chilly water
- 1/4 cup (60 ml) pure maple syrup
- 1/4 cup (60 ml) 100% pure orange juice
- 2 teaspoons lime juice
- 1/4 teaspoon table salt

INSTRUCTIONS

1. Whisk all the ingredients together until completely blended and salt dissolves. Serve immediately. You may also prepare a big quantity ahead of time and store it in an airtight container.
2. Optimal serving temperature is 50°F to 68°F (10°C to 20°C).

NUTRITION

Calories: 98 kcal | Carbohydrates: 24g | Protein: 1g | Fat: 1g | Sodium: 294mg | Potassium: 67mg | Sugar: 20g | Vitamin C: 4.5mg | Calcium: 32mg

---

Low Fodmap Cranberry Cinnamon Swizzle

Serving size: 1 Prep Time 5 mins
Total Time: 5 mins

INGREDIENTS

- 1 tablespoon cranberry juice
- Pinch cinnamon
- 4 ounces (120 ml) ginger ale, ginger beer or ginger sparkling water
- Simple syrup, as requested
- Fresh cranberries & bamboo skewer, optional

INSTRUCTIONS

1. Pour cranberry juice into a glass (we used a champagne glass). Add cinnamon and use anything long and narrow to whisk them together, such a chopstick or long narrow butter knife. Top with ginger beverage and taste.
2. Sweeten with a little Simple Syrup, if desired. Thread a few fresh cranberries on a long bamboo skewer for garnish, if you want. Serve immediately.

NUTRITION

Calories: 48 kcal | Carbohydrates: 12g | Protein: 1g | Fat: 1g | Sodium: 1mg | Sugar: 11g | Vitamin C: 1.4mg

Berry Banana Smoothie

Serving Size: 2
Prep Time: 5 mins

INGREDIENTS

- 1 cup strawberries (hulled)
- 1/2 banana (ripe)
- 1/2 cup blueberries
- 1 cup lactose-free yogurt
- 1 tbsp chia seeds
- 1 cup ice cubes

INSTRUCTIONS

1. Combine strawberries, banana, blueberries, lactose-free yogurt, chia seeds, and ice cubes in a blender.
2. Blend until smooth.
3. Pour into glasses and serve immediately.

NUTRITION

Calories: 150
Protein: 5g, Fat: 6g
Carbohydrates: 20g, Fiber: 5g

Kiwi Spinach Green Smoothie

Serving Size: 2 Prep Time: 7 mins

INGREDIENTS
- 2 kiwis (peeled and sliced)
- 1 cup fresh spinach leaves
- 1/2 cucumber (peeled and sliced)
- 1 cup coconut water
- 1 tablespoon fresh mint leaves
- 1 cup ice cubes

INSTRUCTIONS
1. Combine kiwis, spinach, cucumber, coconut water, mint leaves, and ice cubes in a blender.
2. Blend until smooth.
3. Pour into glasses and serve immediately.

NUTRITION
Calories: 120
Protein: 3g, Fat: 1g
Carbohydrates: 28g, Fiber: 6g

Pineapple Mint Citrus Smoothie

Serving Size: 2 Prep Time: 5 mins

INGREDIENTS

- 1 cup fresh pineapple chunks
- 1/2 orange, peeled and segmented
- 1 tablespoon fresh mint leaves
- 1 cup lactose-free yogurt
- 1 tbsp chia seeds
- 1 cup ice cubes

INSTRUCTIONS

1. Combine pineapple chunks, orange segments, mint leaves, lactose-free yogurt, chia seeds, and ice cubes in a blender.
2. Blend until smooth.
3. Pour into glasses and enjoy!

NUTRITION

Calories: 140
Protein: 5g, Fat: 6g
Carbohydrates: 18g, Fiber: 4g

Raspberry Almond Butter Smoothie

Serving Size: 2 Prep Time: 6 mins

INGREDIENTS

- 1 cup raspberries
- 2 tbsp almond butter
- 1 cup lactose-free milk (or almond milk)
- 1 tbsp chia seeds
- 1 tablespoon maple syrup (optional)
- 1 cup ice cubes

INSTRUCTIONS

Blend raspberries, almond butter, lactose-free milk, chia seeds, maple syrup (if used), and ice cubes until smooth.
Pour into glasses and serve immediately.

NUTRITION

Calories: 220
Protein: 6g, Fat: 12g
Carbohydrates: 24g, Fiber: 8g

Coconut Berry Protein Smoothie

Serving Size: 1 Prep Time: 5 mins

INGREDIENTS
- 1/2 cup mixed berries (strawberries, blueberries, raspberries)
- 1 scoop low FODMAP protein powder
- 1 cup coconut water
- 1 tablespoon shredded coconut
- 1 tbsp chia seeds
- 1 cup ice cubes

INSTRUCTIONS
1. Blend mixed berries, protein powder, coconut water, shredded coconut, chia seeds, and ice cubes until fully incorporated.
2. Pour into glasses and enjoy this protein-packed smoothie!

NUTRITION
Calories: 250
Protein: 20g, Fat: 8g
Carbohydrates: 30g, Fiber: 7g

Mango Passion Fruit Protein Smoothie

Serving Size: 2 Prep Time: 5 mins

INGREDIENTS

- 1 cup fresh mango chunks
- 1 passionfruit, pulp scraped out
- 1 scoop low FODMAP protein powder
- 1 cup lactose-free yogurt
- 1 tbsp chia seeds
- 1 cup ice cubes

INSTRUCTIONS

1. Blend mango chunks, passionfruit pulp, protein powder, lactose-free yogurt, chia seeds, and ice cubes till smooth.
2. Pour into glasses and relish the tropical tastes!

NUTRITION

Calories: 210
Protein: 15g, Fat: 6g
Carbohydrates: 28g, Fiber: 6g

Green Tea Berry Smoothie

Serving Size: 2 Prep Time: 6 mins

INGREDIENTS

- 1 cup mixed berries (strawberries, blueberries, raspberries)
- 1 cup brewed and cooled green tea
- 1 tablespoon fresh mint leaves
- 1 tbsp chia seeds
- 1 tablespoon honey (optional)
- 1 cup ice cubes

INSTRUCTIONS

1. Blend mixed berries, green tea, fresh mint leaves, chia seeds, honey (if used), and ice cubes until nicely integrated.
2. Pour into glasses and enjoy the antioxidant-rich bliss!

NUTRITION

Calories: 110
Protein: 2g, Fat: 2g
Carbohydrates: 22g, Fiber: 6g

Blueberry Banana Oat Smoothie

Serving Size: 2 Prep Time: 7 mins

INGREDIENTS

- 1 cup blueberries
- 1/2 banana (ripe)
- 1/4 cup rolled oats
- 1 cup lactose-free milk
- 1 tbsp almond butter
- 1 cup ice cubes

INSTRUCTIONS

1. Blend blueberries, banana, rolled oats, lactose-free milk, almond butter, and ice cubes until smooth.
2. Pour into glasses and enjoy this nutrient-packed smoothie!

NUTRITION

Calories: 230
Protein: 7g, Fat: 9g
Carbohydrates: 34g, Fiber: 6g

Pineapple Coconut Chia Smoothie

Serving Size: 2 Prep Time: 6 mins

INGREDIENTS

- 1 cup fresh pineapple chunks
- 1/2 cup coconut milk
- 1 tbsp chia seeds
- 1 tablespoon shredded coconut
- 1 tablespoon lime juice
- 1 cup ice cubes

INSTRUCTIONS

1. Blend pineapple chunks, coconut milk, chia seeds, shredded coconut, lime juice, and ice cubes till smooth.
2. Pour into glasses and appreciate the tropical tastes!

NUTRITION

Calories: 180
Protein: 3g, Fat: 12g
Carbohydrates: 18g, Fiber: 6g

Peanut Butter Banana Spinach Smoothie

Serving Size: 2 Prep Time: 8 mins

INGREDIENTS

- 1 banana (ripe)
- 2 tbsp peanut butter
- 1 cup spinach leaves
- 1 cup lactose-free milk
- 1 tbsp chia seeds
- 1 cup ice cubes

INSTRUCTIONS

1. Blend banana, peanut butter, spinach leaves, lactose-free milk, chia seeds, and ice cubes till smooth.
2. Pour into glasses and enjoy this green and protein-packed smoothie!

NUTRITION

Calories: 280
Protein: 11g, Fat: 16g
Carbohydrates: 28g, Fiber: 6g

BONUS 30 DAY MEAL PLAN

Day 1

Breakfast: Scrambled eggs with spinach and tomatoes (cooked in olive oil)
Snack: Greek yogurt with a bunch of strawberries
Lunch: Grilled chicken breast with roasted zucchini and quinoa
Dinner: Baked salmon with steaming green beans and mashed potatoes

---

Day 2

Breakfast: Smoothie with banana, blueberries, lactose-free yogurt, and chia seeds
Snack: Almonds and a tiny orange
Lunch: Turkey and lettuce sandwiches with a side of grapes
Dinner: Shrimp stir-fry with bell peppers, bok choy, and rice

---

Day 3

Breakfast: Omelette with FODMAP-friendly veggies (e.g., bell peppers, spinach, and tomatoes)
Snack: Kiwi slices with lactose-free cottage cheese
Lunch: Quinoa salad with cucumber, cherry tomatoes, and grilled chicken

Dinner: Baked fish with lemon and herbs, served with roasted carrots and green beans

---

Day 4

Breakfast: Overnight oats with lactose-free milk, chia seeds, and strawberries

Snack: Sliced pineapple with a handful of walnuts

Lunch: Spinach and feta omelet with a side of mixed fruit

Dinner: Grilled steak with sweet potato wedges and steamed asparagus

---

Day 5

Breakfast: Banana and blueberry pancakes (using gluten-free flour)

Snack: Lactose-free yogurt with a sprinkling of pumpkin seeds

Lunch: Quinoa dish with grilled shrimp, cucumber, and red pepper

Dinner: Chicken and vegetable curry with basmati rice

Day 6

Breakfast: Smoothie with pineapple, coconut milk, spinach, and chia seeds

Snack: Mixed nuts and a tiny orange

Lunch: Turkey and cranberry wrap with a serving of lactose-free yogurt

Dinner: Baked fish with lemon and dill, served with roasted potatoes and green beans

---

Day 7

Breakfast: Scrambled eggs with sautéed kale and tomatoes

Snack: Grapes with lactose-free cheese cubes

Lunch: Quinoa salad with cherry tomatoes, feta, and grilled chicken

Dinner: Grilled lamb chops with roasted butternut squash and steamed broccoli

---

Day 8

Breakfast: Chia seed pudding with lactose-free milk and kiwi slices

Snack: Almond butter with rice cakes

Lunch: Turkey and avocado salad with mixed greens

Dinner: Baked chicken thighs with lemon and rosemary, served with mashed potatoes and carrots

---

Day 9

Breakfast: Smoothie bowl with banana, blueberries, and gluten-free granola

Snack: Mixed nuts and grapes
Lunch: Tuna salad with lettuce, cucumber, and olives
Dinner: Grilled swordfish with a side of quinoa and steamed asparagus

---

Day 10

Breakfast: Omelette with FODMAP-friendly veggies and lactose-free cheese
Snack: Pineapple slices with a handful of walnuts
Lunch: Shrimp and vegetable stir-fry with rice
Dinner: Baked cod with a side of roasted sweet potatoes and green beans

---

Day 11

Breakfast: Peanut butter and banana smoothie with lactose-free yogurt and a sprinkling of chia seeds
Snack: Hard-boiled eggs with grape tomatoes
Lunch: Grilled chicken Caesar salad with lactose-free Caesar dressing
Dinner: Baked fish with a dill and lemon sauce, paired with roasted Brussels sprouts and quinoa

---

Day 12

Breakfast: Blueberry and coconut milk overnight oats with a handful of raspberries

Snack: Mixed almonds and kiwi slices
Lunch: Turkey and Swiss cheese roll-ups with a side of cucumber slices
Dinner: Stir-fried tofu with bok choy, carrots, and rice noodles

---

Day 13

Breakfast: Spinach and feta crustless quiche with cherry tomatoes
Snack: Rice cakes with smoked fish and lemon
Lunch: Quinoa dish with roasted eggplant, cherry tomatoes, and grilled chicken
Dinner: Baked fish with a tomato and olive salsa, served with steaming green beans and quinoa

---

Day 14

Breakfast: Raspberry and almond milk smoothie with a scoop of low FODMAP protein powder
Snack: Carrot sticks with lactose-free cream cheese
Lunch: Shrimp and avocado lettuce wraps with a side of grapes
Dinner: Grilled pork chops with a mustard and rosemary marinade, served with mashed sweet potatoes and sautéed spinach

---

Day 15

Breakfast: Chia seed pudding with lactose-free milk, topped with sliced kiwi

Snack: Mixed berries with a handful of walnuts

Lunch: Quinoa salad with cucumber, cherry tomatoes, and canned tuna

Dinner: Baked chicken thighs with a lemon and thyme glaze, followed with roasted butternut squash and green beans

Day 16

Breakfast: Banana and almond butter smoothie with lactose-free yogurt and a sprinkling of chia seeds

Snack: Sliced oranges with a handful of macadamia nuts

Lunch: Turkey and cranberry quinoa bowl with mixed greens

Dinner: Baked fish in a lemon and dill sauce, paired with roasted sweet potatoes and steamed broccoli

Day 17

Breakfast: Blueberry and pecan granola with lactose-free milk

Snack: Greek yogurt with a handful of raspberries

Lunch: Chicken and vegetable stir-fry with low FODMAP stir-fry sauce and jasmine rice

Dinner: Grilled swordfish with a lime and cilantro marinade, complemented with quinoa and sautéed asparagus

---

Day 18

Breakfast: Spinach and tomato frittata with lactose-free cheese

Snack: Carrot sticks with hummus

Lunch: Shrimp and avocado salad with mixed greens and a lemon vinaigrette

Dinner: Baked chicken drumsticks with a low FODMAP BBQ sauce, paired with mashed potatoes and green beans

---

Day 19

Breakfast: Pineapple and coconut milk smoothie with a handful of spinach

Snack: Mixed berries with a dollop of lactose-free yogurt

Lunch: Quinoa and veggie filled bell peppers with ground turkey

Dinner: Grilled lamb kebabs with a mint and lemon marinade, complemented with rice and roasted Brussels sprouts

---

Day 20

Breakfast: Chia seed and strawberry parfait with lactose-free yogurt
Snack: Kiwi slices with a handful of walnuts
Lunch: Turkey and Swiss cheese roll-ups with a side of mixed fruit
Dinner: Baked salmon with a mustard and dill glaze, served with quinoa and sautéed spinach

---

Day 21
Breakfast: Smoothie bowl with mixed berries, lactose-free yogurt, and a sprinkling of pumpkin seeds
Snack: Hard-boiled eggs with grape tomatoes
Lunch: Quinoa and chicken salad with cherry tomatoes, cucumber, and a low FODMAP vinaigrette
Dinner: Baked fish with a ginger and soy marinade, served with jasmine rice and steamed broccoli

---

Day 22
Breakfast: Banana and raspberry oatmeal (using gluten-free oats) with a sprinkle of maple syrup
Snack: Mixed nuts and a tiny orange
Lunch: Turkey and cranberry lettuce wraps with a side of cucumber slices

Dinner: Grilled shrimp skewers with a lemon and herb marinade, complemented with quinoa and roasted Brussels sprouts

---

Day 23

Breakfast: Spinach and feta breakfast burrito with a side of grapes

Snack: Carrot sticks with lactose-free cream cheese

Lunch: Quinoa and vegetable stir-fry with tofu and a low FODMAP stir-fry sauce

Dinner: Baked chicken thighs with a rosemary and lemon glaze, served with mashed sweet potatoes and green beans

---

Day 24

Breakfast: Pineapple and coconut chia pudding with lactose-free milk

Snack: Rice cakes with smoked fish and lemon

Lunch: Shrimp and avocado quinoa dish with mixed greens and a lime vinaigrette

Dinner: Grilled pork chops with a mustard and thyme marinade, complemented with roasted butternut squash and sautéed spinach

---

Day 25

Breakfast: Blueberry and almond milk smoothie with a scoop of low FODMAP protein powder
Snack: Greek yogurt with a handful of raspberries
Lunch: Chicken and vegetable curry with basmati rice
Dinner: Baked fish with a tomato and olive salsa, served with rice and steamed asparagus

---

Day 26

Breakfast: Banana and blueberry pancakes (using gluten-free flour) with a side of strawberries
Snack: Mixed almonds and kiwi slices
Lunch: Turkey and Swiss cheese roll-ups with a serving of lactose-free yogurt
Dinner: Baked chicken drumsticks in a rosemary and lemon marinade, served with mashed potatoes and green beans

---

Day 27

Breakfast: Spinach and tomato frittata with lactose-free cheese
Snack: Sliced oranges with a handful of macadamia nuts
Lunch: Quinoa and veggie filled bell peppers with ground turkey

Dinner: Grilled swordfish with a lime and cilantro marinade, complemented with quinoa and sautéed asparagus

---

Day 28

Breakfast: Pineapple and coconut milk smoothie with a handful of spinach
Snack: Hard-boiled eggs with grape tomatoes
Lunch: Turkey and avocado lettuce sandwiches with a side of mixed fruit
Dinner: Baked fish with a tomato and olive salsa, served with steaming green beans and quinoa

---

Day 29

Breakfast: Chia seed and strawberry parfait with lactose-free yogurt
Snack: Mixed berries with a dollop of lactose-free yogurt
Lunch: Quinoa and chicken salad with cherry tomatoes, cucumber, and a low FODMAP vinaigrette
Dinner: Grilled lamb kebabs with a mint and lemon marinade, complemented with rice and roasted Brussels sprouts

---

Day 30

Breakfast: Smoothie bowl with mixed berries, lactose-free yogurt, and a sprinkling of pumpkin seeds

Snack: Sliced strawberries with lactose-free cottage cheese

Lunch: Grilled shrimp skewers with a lemon and herb marinade, complemented with quinoa and roasted Brussels sprouts

Dinner: Baked fish with a ginger and soy marinade, served with jasmine rice and steamed broccoli

Conclusion

In conclusion, this cookbook on the low FODMAP diet is a valuable resource for individuals wanting to enhance their general well-being and manage the digestive troubles that they are experiencing. This cookbook enables you to take charge of your health and enjoy a broad range of flavorful meals without provoking unpleasant symptoms by presenting recipes that are not only delicious and Healthy also simple to follow and correspond to the recommendations for low FODMAP diets. If you have the correct information and resources, adopting a diet that is low in FODMAPs may be a lifestyle change that is not only beneficial to your digestive health but also pleasurable. This alteration can also improve your quality of life.

Appendix

Dear Readers,

By means of this cookbook, I would like to convey my deepest appreciation for your decision to go on a journey of discovery with me into the realm of low FODMAP cookery. Your encouragement and excitement mean the world to me, and I really hope that the recipes and knowledge included within these pages offer you happiness, sustenance, and comfort.

I am writing to respectfully request that you give some thought to providing an honest comment or review of the book if you have a minute. Your comments not only assist me in becoming a better writer and creator, but they also play a significant part in increasing the exposure of the book, which leads to an increase in the number of people who are able to learn about the advantages of following a diet low in FODMAPs.

Again, I want to express my gratitude for your participation in this adventure. Your assistance is much valued and appreciated.

ENJOY YOUR MEALS